DIARY OF A

MEDICAL NIGHTMARE

Annette Stremecki

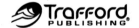

www.trafford.com

North America & international
toll-free: 1 888 232 4444 (USA & Canada)
phone: 250 383 6864 ♦ fax: 250 383 6804
email: info@trafford.com

The United Kingdom & Europe
phone: +44 (0)1865 722 113 ♦ local rate: 0845 230 9601
facsimile: +44 (0)1865 722 868 ♦ email: info.uk@trafford.com

10 9 8 7 6 5 4 3 2

DEDICATION

With love, I dedicate this book to...

my loving husband Ken. Without you, this book would not have happened. We make one heck of a team. Thank you for holding my hand.

my wonderful children and grandchildren; Robert, his wife Lorena and their sons Daniel and Marc; Joanne, her husband Dennis and their sons Nicolas and Luc; Rachelle, her husband Jed and their children Tristan, Tahlia and "Baby" Cayden. You are all such great gifts! I feel so blessed to have been given the opportunity to be your mother and grandmother. Your love has given me strength and courage. I love you very much.

my sisters Terry and Michelle, my brother Bernie, and their families. Thank you for all your help, prayers and understanding.

my father Philippe, mother Judith and sister May, in heaven, who taught me about courage, patience, love and miracles.

my dear friend Elaine; no matter what, you embrace life to the fullest. You're an inspiration!

ACKNOWLEDGEMENTS

With gratitude, I want to acknowledge my extended family, dear and amazing friends, neighbors and co-workers who were always there for me. You know who you are. Thank you for your help and continuous support.

To Gerda, Hélène and Sharon, my chronic fatigue/ fibromyalgia friends who have "walked in my shoes" and know exactly what I am talking about. Thank you, my prayers are with you.

I thank Mr. James Ludwar for his sound legal advice and for being such a kind and understanding person.

Thank you to Dr. Andrew Sereda for finally identifying my illness and giving us hope; Drs. Trethart and Sandhar for your direction and help; Dr. Hasik for your amazing chiropractic care and for setting me straight. Dr. Warness, for your help; and, Dr. Stan Gerhart for always "lending me an ear" and for teaching me about the wonders of energy testing. You are all such understanding doctors and have made such a difference in the quality of my life. Thank you for furthering your education to include non-conventional and/or preventative medicine.

My thanks to the various healthcare practitioners, such as chiropractors, reflexologists, reiki therapists, therapeutic massage therapists, etc. What rewarding and helpful work you do.

Heartfelt thanks to Dr. Bernie Siegel for teaching me about body and mind communication through his book "Peace, Love and Healing."

To all the "conventional" medical doctors who were and are genuinely concerned. Thank you for your help and dedication.

May you all work together in harmony for the betterment of mankind.

Above all, I thank God, my strength and savior, for his unconditional love.

FORWARD

Not until serious illness is experienced personally, does one fully understand the devastation it can bring. Or, the enormous need for understanding, support, help, determination, faith and love.

My illness has given me the opportunity to learn like I have never yet learned. It now seems that it must have come my way as a teacher enabling me to help others through my experience.

My book is not intended to be a great literary work. It is only a shared experience in my life, written by an ordinary woman. Please forgive any errors in spelling and grammar.

For you, "My Story."

Note: The names of doctors and medical institutions have been changed to fictitious names, except those in the acknowledgments. Any fictitious name picked that may be the name of a real person or institution is strictly coincidental.

Spring 1983

Spring, a time of renewal and new beginnings—that's what it was for me also. After a difficult divorce, I met a wonderful man, had learned to love and laugh again and life was enjoyable.

We had recently moved into our new home and I had a job with a major school system. Also, our department had moved into the renovated wing of a school and I had my own office. The challenge was high but it was great.

My children, Robert (23), Joanne (20) and Rachelle (9), were like a natural spring to me. They provided me with refreshing memories, opportunity for enjoyment of their many talents and were constant reminders of never-ending unconditional love.

Driving to work one beautiful early spring morning, I was thinking how lucky I was. As I crossed an overpass, I became dizzy and started going to the right. It was momentary and a most frightening experience. I thought jokingly that, if I didn't know better, I was pregnant. It would have taken a miracle, as I had a hysterectomy about 6 years ago. I shrugged it off as an after effect of a flu I recently had. As the weeks passed, it didn't leave me. In addition to the dizziness, I had headaches, felt tired and was generally ill. My many activities were put on hold. No longer could I play tennis, jog or ride my bike with my family. I couldn't believe how tired I was!

Sitting down and seriously evaluating what was happening, I concluded it must be due to all the stress and changes I had been through. It had to be that! I resolved to try and change my lifestyle and rest more. I had the summer off and for a time I felt a bit better.

In September I returned to work thinking that I would also like to take another university course this year. That thought was short lived when I became worse again. This kept on all through the winter of 83/84. It was getting most alarming. All that winter my general practitioner could not come up with an answer and concluded it was stress.

Spring 1984
The dizziness got much worse so I again made an appointment with my general practitioner. He was not in; therefore, I was booked with another doctor. After talking with her and sharing what I had been experiencing, she suggested I see a neurologist. I was booked for a consultation and an electronystagmography (ENG). The test would not be pleasant, however, it could give us answers that we needed. The test consisted of flooding the ears with water at various temperatures. He indicated that he felt it might be Meniere's disease, a balance disorder. He thought that the symptoms should leave me but it was unpredictable as to when the attacks would again occur, if indeed it were Meniere's disease.

In addition, I made an appointment with an ear, nose and throat (ENT) specialist who had taken out my tonsils about 15 years earlier. After a hearing test, he indicated that my hearing had deteriorated somewhat bilaterally and agreed that my problems were most likely related to Meniere's disease.

The symptoms continued along with severe headaches. I returned to see the female general practitioner that had referred me to the neurologist. This time she referred me to another neurologist, as the one that I saw previously had become very ill and could no longer practice.

From the first meeting with this neurologist, I felt indifference and coldness. I was most uncomfortable with him and felt I was imposing on his time. After a few visits he ordered skull films and a cranial CAT scan. As indicated in his report (I will share with you later how I came to be in possession of this and other reports), he felt the CAT scan was normal, although it did indicate upbeat nystagmus suggesting involvement of central mechanisms. When I read this report it was like a foreign language to me. It was never mentioned or explained to me. The radiologist's report indicated I had left the hospital without being discharged, which was not so. After sitting there for about an hour, I had asked the nurse if I was now able to leave and she had said, "I don't see why not."

During the follow-up meeting, I was told that the CAT scan was completely normal and that my headaches were probably migraine in nature and that I looked "anxious." I replied that if he had my symptoms, I imagined he would also feel anxious. That was probably the wrong thing to say but no doubt true.

The symptoms continued on and off that spring. At times it seemed like they might stop, only to start again. As summer approached, we were busy planning Robert's wedding. Like last summer, I seemed to improve slightly. The wedding was beautiful and it was nice visiting with all the relatives. The summer went by with some of the dizziness occurring, but mostly when I was very tired.

3

Fall 1984

I returned to work all excited. Ken and I had decided to marry that December. We started making plans. It was to be a small family wedding. At times that fall my symptoms seemed worse. I tried not to mention them to anyone. I thought, "If I don't talk or think about them, they might just go away." Was it psychological? Was I more stressed out than I thought?

In October 1984, I went to do an errand during my lunch-hour. It was a lovely fall day and I looked forward to the drive. As I drove back to my office, I approached a traffic circle and saw an elderly woman step off the curb in front of the half-ton truck in front of me. I heard the shriek of brakes and I put on my brakes as an older green car swerved from the wrong incoming lane to my right and crossed between the truck and my car. I could not believe I hadn't hit him. As my car stopped, I was hit from behind with incredible force. I remember lifting my head from the steering wheel and shutting the car off. I was shaking and remember screaming when I was hit. My leg hurt and I seemed to be in a fog. The top of the dash had flown over my head and was in the back seat, as were my briefcase, purse and sunglasses. I heard the driver of the truck that had hit me saying, "Are you all right?" He kept repeating this over and over. I managed to answer that I thought I was but was not sure. "Please call the police," I said. I was very dizzy and sore. I noticed a car stop and saw it was my department superintendent and his assistant. They asked if they could call Ken and I was thankful for their help. The police arrived, asked some questions and then took me to

4

the Layco Hospital. I was looked at and given a neck collar for whiplash and released. The doctor told me to take it easy as I may have suffered a concussion because I had blacked out. The policeman called it a no-fault accident, as he felt it was due to the elderly lady suddenly deciding to cross at a no-cross walk before looking for traffic. It was a shame that I was so shaken and confused at the time or, I would have asked him why two vehicles managed to stop and the third didn't when he was much further away. The car was a wreck! It was only a few years old so we decided we should have it fixed, but it never was the same.

I wore the collar and had physiotherapy for a few weeks. Because I was so busy at work, I only took a few days off. I continued to have dizziness, headaches and now had back pain with it. Not having much patience with illness, I tried mild exercise. I was convinced this was a bad time I was going through and it would pass.

The next year was an adjustment for all of us with its expected ups and downs. My health remained about the same. A lot more of my time was spent going to doctors than I appreciated. I had the flu again and felt awful. Shortly thereafter, I experienced severe chest pain and my eldest daughter Joanne called an ambulance. I was given an electrocardiogram (ECG) and given a prescription for Tylenol with Codeine. During that emergency visit, I mentioned the persistent bladder and yeast infections that I was constantly battling (this I had mentioned before to the general practitioners). The Tylenol with Codeine had caused rapid heartbeat and chest pain and I was once again taken to emergency by a co-worker. I was told I had an allergy to

Codeine and to never take it again, as the reactions were severe.

That summer Joanne was married and looked so beautiful in her white gown. Robert, Lorena and Rachelle were all in the bridal party. They looked so nice and I was so proud of them all. Again it was a beautiful wedding and a special time with family and friends.

In December 1985, after having seen an urologist, I was booked for a cystoscopy (a bladder stretch and scraping). This seemed to help the urgency to urinate, but I still woke up with a headache when I had a full bladder. Because I was not easily discouraged, I thought, "This will all pass, my health will return." But this was not to be, and so began a "medical nightmare" that would last for years.

December 1985

Ken came home with a dozen roses; we were celebrating our first anniversary. It was to be a special weekend. Saturday, December 28 I woke up and told Ken to sleep, that I would get up and do a little ironing and make breakfast. As I turned to get up, the room began to spin and I felt like I would fly off the bed. I blacked out for a few minutes and as I came to, I lost control of my bowels. I was so embarrassed! Ken called an ambulance and I was brought to the Humanity Hospital. We told the doctor that I had been diagnosed as possibly having Meniere's disease, so an ENT specialist was called in. The neurologist I had seen previously was called, but his assisting student saw me. I was hospitalized for what was thought to be a severe Meniere's disease attack. By the fifth day it was obvious it was not simply a Meniere's disease attack, as I was still dizzy and would fall to the right when I tried to walk. On the sixth day I was told that it was probably (that famous word) a brain stem virus and it would take time to get better. Viral tests were not done at that time, nor was an infection specialist consulted.

That experience in the hospital was far from pleasant. I had to share a room with another patient. The first patient coughed for 2 days and nights. When they moved her, I was told she had pneumonia. Poor her, it was not her fault. The next lady was a disabled person in for abdominal surgery. She was unpleasant to the staff and even worse with me. She was moved after 3 days. The following lady had emphysema and was furious at being hospitalized. She threw things around and swore incredibly when she was at the sink clearing out her phlegm. Must I elaborate any further? I asked for a wheelchair and called Ken. I told him that I was going to ask to be discharged, as nothing was being done for me and I wasn't sure that I could face another roommate at this time. Even my usual sense of humor had now vanished completely.

Our first anniversary was spent with Ken and the children sitting by my bedside. Guilty feelings were setting in. How could I spoil such a special time? What had poor Ken married? This was not the person he met 4 years ago.

I was discharged after 10 long days and told to book an appointment with the ENT clinic in 3 weeks. "Why that clinic, if it's not Meniere's disease?" I thought. Although I was incapacitated when released, the report read: After the investigations, the patient felt well and was discharged on January 5, 1986 to her home in good condition. How can they have written outright lies? Self-protection I imagine. There should be a law that allows patients, or next of kin, to read medical reports and question their contents, if they so wish. It is absolutely incredible what goes on behind the scene regarding patients.

On the way home we shared that the news about a possible virus was better than of having Meniere's disease. A virus might just go away. The 3 weeks at home were spent hoping for improvement. I contacted work with no specific news as to when I could return. I went slowly from one chair to the next and down the stairs from our bedroom while stopping and sitting on each step. My mother came to help and keep me company. Her kindness and help was much appreciated. I could not believe what was happening and what I was doing to Ken and my family.

By the time the appointment came, I couldn't wait to see what they would do to help me. At this time I was barely able to walk. We felt this situation simply had to improve; it had gone on long enough. I was given another hearing test. I was not told why it had to be repeated so soon. My expectations for some indication of what was ravaging my body and positive direction were not to be. We were told, "Be patient now, these things take time." What things? I wanted to know. Was it still a virus? Did I indeed have Meniere's disease? The questions could not be answered at this time we were told. How sad to waste Health Care money and devastate people in such a fashion. We returned home feeling worse than when we left.

I was more determined than ever to find answers and get help. My conclusion, at this time, was that so far the doctors were not looking at this in a serious way. I was somehow getting the feeling that being 43 years old and female was not helping matters. My plan of action was to find a doctor that would be willing to get to the bottom of things. I then decided to make an appointment with a general practitioner I knew personally. He would surely know this was serious and provide me with help. Having known I had been through marital stressful times, he quickly concluded it was stress and that it could bring on all kinds of problems. I could not dispute that fact and after a long talk, I was convinced he was right. He prescribed all kinds of medication and told me to return in about a month. After picking up my medication, I left for home determined this would surely do the trick.

At this point, I would like to share with you that I had never taken medication unless it was absolutely necessary. I looked at all these pills and thought, "Okay, this is absolutely necessary, I have to do something." I decided to only take half the recommended dosage, as I knew I was highly sensitive to medication. The side effects were terrible! I felt I was in a fog and had chest pains and personality changes. I also felt nauseous. Absolutely nothing was improving with this medication, except I was now dealing with added things. I stopped taking them, as I didn't need additional symptoms to deal with.

On January 18, I woke up with numbness in both arms and some in the left side of my face and both legs. Now what was happening? Would it ever end? I made another appointment with the neurologist and told him what had happened. This time he seemed a little more concerned and sympathetic. He did not find anything of significance during the examination. He thought that most of the symptoms were related to anxiety and told me to take 1 mg of Ativan before going to sleep and report any changes to him. I took the Ativan as prescribed, but found I had to cut the dose in half because of side effects. It was a relief to sleep better as I also had started pain in my muscles and it would keep me awake. Although I slept better, my symptoms persisted.

I returned on February 7, 1986, to see the same neurologist. He decided it was time to have more tests done. He booked the following tests with another specialist: a visual evoke response, a brain stem auditory evoke response and a somatosensory evoke response. In addition, a spine x-ray was taken; an ECG and blood work was done. At this time my symptoms were: numbness; pain and tightness in the chest, left side of neck, arms and left shoulder; headaches and upset stomach. I was very weak and tired and had tremors in my hands and legs. I had trouble doing certain tasks, such as lifting a pitcher and pouring. Devastated, I prayed that this would end and an answer to what was invading my body. I also asked to be referred to a specialist in infectious diseases. This appointment was set up for March 5, 1986.

The infectious disease specialist explained that it was too late for the viral tests because I had been ill for so long. After the exam, he explained that he felt I might be suffering from more than one condition and that I maybe dealing with the after effects of a viral infection. I was hopeful that someone might understand what was happening to me. He indicated he would suggest a spinal tap and CAT scan of the upper back. His assistant agreed that these tests might give some answers (they were never done). I'm not aware what suggestions were made to the neurologist or whether he decided against them. I can imagine the picture that I painted at this time. They must have thought I was a neurotic middle-aged lady. I had always been intimidated by doctors and was taught they should be placed on a pedestal, as they knew everything. This I was finding out was not the case. They are human beings like all of us and do not necessarily know everything. In fact, I felt that the medical profession had a lot to learn!

On March 8, 1986, I went to see my eye doctor. He, at that time, found convergence in the left eye and asked if I had been checked for multiple sclerosis (MS). This took me by surprise because not that long before my gynecologist had asked me the same question. I replied I had tests done recently and I would see the neurologist and have the results shortly.

During the third week in March, I experienced three severe attacks. The first was a shooting pain from the upper right side of my back going all the way down to the right heel and back up into my neck. The second was the same severe shooting pain through my upper left arm and the third had the same severity and went through the left side of my head. These attacks occurred about 3 days apart at which time I was doing nothing different or strenuous. Each time the attacks left me completely drained and the pain took a long time to subside.

My next appointment with the neurologist was booked for March 21, 1986. By this time I knew something was very wrong with me and that getting answers wouldn't come easy for us. Things were getting strained. Without straight answers, it would be impossible to collect long-term disability benefits. We were all finding this so hard to cope with. The children and family were worried. Rachelle was only 11 and couldn't understand why the doctors weren't helping her mom get better. As much as we tried to hide it from family and friends, it was impossible to do so. We had our faith and prayed that somehow we would get help. Philippe, my Dad who is in heaven, had taught me love, humor, love of music, courage and strength. Without these important teachings, I would have lost hope. Somehow we drank in everything and anything that was funny and happy. It was like having a bank of good things we could draw from to help us cope.

During my examination on March 21, the neurologist found that again his examination was normal, except for extreme tenderness in the thoracic paraspinal muscles all the way down my spine. At that time, my back was so sore I could not lean back on anything hard. It was also swollen along the spine. The neurologist felt that further tests were not necessary at this time. We asked about a second neurological opinion and were advised against this. He suggested a psychiatric opinion be considered and perhaps a trial of antidepressants should be tried. I left for home thinking I must be going crazy.

Back I went to my general practitioner and asked him for a referral to another neurologist. He insisted it was stress and said, "If you want to get better, you have to stay on your stress medication." Ken and I were at our wits' end. I was so sore, fatigued and frustrated that we decided to go to the Hope Clinic in another country. If we couldn't get answers here, we would get them elsewhere. We arranged to have Joanne and Dennis stay with Rachelle. How I hated to leave her, but every time I thought of my husband and children, it made me want to get answers all the more.

April 1986

We had set up a bed in our mini van for me. We cried as we watched Rachelle run beside the van, crying and shouting, "I love you Mom." This was to be an expensive trip, which we really couldn't afford.

As we drove, Ken had to be ever so careful as every bump hurt me. We drove as far as we could that day. I remember that as we drove past the community center of a small town, Ken noticed they were having a flea market. He said, "Let's stop for a few minutes." Knowing how he loved them, I told him to stop. He helped me out of the van and held me as we walked towards the door. I was so tired and sore I had to return to the van. I was in tears. I told Ken to go back without me. Memories flooded back to the times when we had hunted for treasures at flea markets and second hand stores. I wondered if I would ever be able to do that again. We continued driving until we arrived at a major city, where we stayed the night.

Eventually, after what seemed like an eternity (4 days), we arrived at our destination. For convenience, we took a motel a few blocks away from the clinic. The next day we registered at the Hope Clinic. We were told that I would be considered a priority patient and would get the first available cancellation, as we did not have an appointment. After 7 agonizing days, I got my appointment. I was given information and directed to a consultant who would see me first. After listening to what had been happening to me, he informed me that I would first be going through tests like regular blood chemistry, urinalysis, cholesterol, thyroxin, pap smear etc., etc. One morning I was booked for a test before breakfast and as I waited, I fainted. I was put in a wheelchair and an appointment was made with my consultant. He suggested I be hospitalized, but indicated I would be under the services of doctors in the hospital. I was torn; we liked this doctor and were hesitant to continue under new ones. I had little choice but to go into the hospital. I was so ill, seemed much worse in the morning and my symptoms were many. I felt partial paralysis in my left side and had incredible headaches. My whole body was sore and I felt dizzy and weak. In addition to this, we were frustrated and anxious to get help and answers.

Once admitted, my vital signs were taken for the first 5 days. At that time, MS was suspected. Many of the doctors were indifferent and I missed the caring consultant I had started with. I was lucky to have a young intern called Dr. Ring assigned to my case. He was most supportive and encouraging. After a few days I started to feel that some of the doctors were questioning what I was telling them. Physical therapy was started for what they felt was fibrositis. Also, I was given a psychological test. Let me share with you how this instrument was presented to me.

Ken, as faithful as ever, was sitting by my bed. A nurse walked in and put what appeared to be a questionnaire on my table saying, "Please complete this." Having worked in evaluation for a number of years, I quickly concluded this was a psychological evaluation of some kind. As I started to complete the questionnaire, I thought, "Okay I'll do anything to get answers and get well." At this time, remember that I was scared, frustrated and stressed from all the tests I was going through, lonesome for home, etc. I started the questionnaire and about half way through I asked Ken to help me complete it as I was so tired and everything was getting blurry. He knew me as well as anybody. Although we weren't told what it was and why I had to do this, I had gathered the answers quickly. Little did we know, however, that this test would be a thorn in my life for years.

The next day Mr. Psychiatrist, along with two interns (bodyguards we called them), came into my room. I will never forget what he looked like. Like an eagle about to attack! You would have thought they were attending a funeral the way they looked and talked. Actually, it was difficult to keep from smiling as the poor doctor looked like he needed help rather than me. He said, "I hear they're going ahead with the magnetic resonance imagery (MRI) test. That's the ultimate test you know, they can't do too much more after that." As they left, I thought, "Please God keep his kind away from me." Needless to elaborate, my first experience with a psychiatrist was not good. I was to find out later that they are not all like this. When we later looked at our statement, we were astounded to see that the charge for those few minutes of consultation was $150.

We were told the MRI report was within the normal range. They had detected narrowing in the cervical area of the spine and in the esophagus, but explained these findings should not cause all the symptoms I was experiencing. Dr. Ring explained that this test eliminated MS by about 90%.

Rachelle's birthday was on May 10 and I wanted to be there for it. At this point we were told I might as well go home as so many tests had been done and nothing significant had been detected. The night before I left, Dr. Ring stayed up most of the night researching my case. He shared with us he still thought there was something that might have been missed. He concluded I really was ill, but it had to be something new that they were not aware of yet. Since my muscles were so sore, an exercise program was developed for me. It was noted on this program that I had fibrositis. Before I left, the psychiatrist came by and explained how we sometimes "carry these things on in an imaginary way" and asked me to follow this up back home. This took less than 5 minutes, nothing more was said. As he left the room with his two bodyguards (they never spoke once), I felt sorry for him, he never once smiled, nor had a kind word for me.

I left May 14, 1986, from the hospital for home. I had missed Rachelle's birthday. Our hopes were up, nothing serious had been detected. With rest and exercise I would surely get better soon. "Fibrositis," we wondered, "What would the insurance company think of that diagnosis?" I was not aware that something like fibrositis could devastate a body so much. I was determined to do my own research regarding this. I was told a report would be sent to my general practitioner.

It felt so good to be home at last. Although I still had my symptoms, Ken and I were convinced I would soon find my health again. After all, a major clinic had not found anything considered serious. The fibrositis would go, as well as everything else. It would just take a little time and I would be "myself" again.

June 1986

For about 3 weeks in June my vertigo left me. During this time I experienced severe headaches unequal to any I previously had. Constant hot flashes and perspiration were added to my list of symptoms. Since I had a hysterectomy approximately 8 years before, I suspected these new symptoms might have something to do with hormones. I made an appointment with my gynecologist. I was not given any blood work for hormonal levels. He simply suggested I talk to my general practitioner. Having known my recent history and the fact that I had recently come back from a major health clinic, he seemed to think that if anything was wrong they would have detected it. How disheartened I felt as I left. Was I destined to spend half of my time sitting in doctors' offices trying to get answers? Would I lose my determination and just give up to be an invalid with a disease that had no name?

My life that summer was a shamble. Trying to hide my pain did not work well. I rested, watched my diet, tried to walk a bit and did all the exercises suggested by the Hope Clinic. In August 1986, I experienced vertigo again, back pain, pain in the shoulders and upper arms, pain in the neck (in more ways than one), headaches, intermittent numbness in my left hand and extreme fatigue. I felt bloated, had trouble digesting, had night sweats and my hands and feet were red and swollen.

I had managed to collect a few months of disability benefits with great frustration caused by the insurance company. Only when a person tries to collect, do they see the true picture of these companies. It is all fine and dandy to give them money on a monthly basis, but to get some back is a totally different story. I made a decision to try going back to work, at least part-time. If I could focus on something else, my health might improve. I was thankful my department superintendent agreed to let me try to see if I could cope. Furthermore, I would be rid of the insurance people.

Working again proved more difficult than I imagined. Trying to focus on my work was difficult with the constant pain. Psychologically, however, it did help. The one thing that scared me was that I noticed I was not as "sharp," as usual. My memory was bad and I had to look up things I once had at the tip of my fingers. Towards mid afternoon I was so fatigued, I could have dropped right where I was.

By December 1986, in addition to the other symptoms, I had pain in my left arm and both legs almost constantly. My left leg was swelling so that I had trouble walking. One morning I looked at myself in the mirror and thought, "Who are you?" The person looking back was not me. I seemed like a stranger. I could not believe what had happened and was still happening. I was so frustrated and mad I just about lost it and broke the mirror. This would not help matters; I had to talk myself back to sanity. I could allow myself my crying sessions but I could not let this lead me to insanity. I would keep going—I would win this war!

Once again I made another appointment with my general practitioner. He told me, "Now, don't let this get to you. Try to rest a little more and come back in a few weeks and we'll talk again." Was I going mad? Of course not, something was ravaging my body, but what? I would keep searching no matter what. I had too much to live for. "Think back," I thought, "there must be someone who is willing to listen."

I still had my appointment with the infectious disease specialist for December 15. By this time I was developing a phobia about going to hospitals and doctors. Only the fact that I had to find answers, kept me going to them. He seemed genuinely concerned as I attempted to explain to him what was happening to me. He asked me questions and checked me. I was asked to do 10 sit-ups so he could check my heart. These were hard to do because of the pain. He explained to me that because of the shortness of breath and other symptoms he would prescribe Nitroglycerine until I could see a cardiologist on January 30, 1987.

Christmas has always been a special time for me. This one was no exception even if I had a monster ravaging my body. I could now only dream of the times I would rush around doing the shopping, baking and caroling with our friends, etc. This year I needed more help than ever. These were times where I had to play the hardest role ever. It seemed impossible at times but I tried my best. So many times I cried silently and prayed I would get through the day without showing my pain and discomfort. If it was frustrating for me, it must have been even more so for Ken and my family. The guilt associated with this monstrous situation was increasing. I could feel my mental state deteriorating. This was hard to face, as I have always considered myself the strong one in the family, able to help others and cope with difficulties. I looked at my family and our Christmas tree that year and wondered if it would be the last Christmas I would be with the ones I loved so dearly.

January 1987

A New Year begins! The beginning of a New Year has always been a time of planning and of looking forward with determination. I decided this year would be no exception; in fact, I was filled with hope on this New Year Day. One way or another, I would win this battle. As I found out, I would have to work on this determination. On January 7 I felt worse when I went to bed and woke up later with severe pain in my chest and left arm. I took a "Nitro" and we went to the Humanity Hospital. After a long night in emergency, I was admitted for further investigation under the head internal medicine specialist. A senior resident was assigned to my case, as well as, another resident doctor. The hospital I was in is a teaching hospital; therefore, I was examined and questioned by many doctors. We told the doctor who was in charge of my case about the Hope Clinic, as we felt he should know everything. He said, "It seems to me if there was something wrong with you they would have found out what it was." Ken and I looked at each other and instantly knew what he thought. Only a few months before, I had heard the same thing from my gynecologist. I was then put through more tests—blood work, ECG, echocardiogram (a cardiac ultrasound), etc. I could not make the stress test as I fainted that morning. I was told I would be moved to the Internal Medicine unit.

Ken and the children came to visit often. It hurt me so to see them so concerned about this ongoing illness. I was also worried about my work situation. How long would they hold my position for me? Would I even have a job to go back to? Little did we know, how long I would be in the hospital. It's a good thing God has arranged it so we can't tell the future. At this time, I'll continue to write in my diary about my hospital stay on a daily-basis for the benefit of those who can learn from what occurred.

January 10, 1987

Today I had blood work done and an ECG also. I was given "Nitro" before the test. I had upper back pain, pain in my left arm, leg cramps, numbness in my left hand, heart palpitations and pain in my chest. My family was here to see me. I'm worried about Ken; he looks so tired and pale. How can I do this to him?

January 11, 1987

Today is Sunday and I don't feel able to go to the chapel. I looked at our acreage house plans, a dream that we were trying to follow through with. Even trying to concentrate on these was too tiring. Around noon I had a fainting spell. Shortly after, the doctor was in and said my ECG was normal. The day is long here. Ken came to see me at 3 p.m. This is teaching me how important it is to visit people who are ill. It is such good therapy to see Ken, family and friends. Ken and I talked about our acreage and how I would get well and we would have a wonderful life there. As he tries to encourage me, I feel so sick that I think I will never see those times. He stayed until 8 p.m. and it was so hard to see him go. I'm scarred and lonely and ask God to be with me and help me. I try to sleep, but I'm so sore I can't.

January 12, 1987

Blood tests are taken again. I'm weighed and can't believe how I've gained weight, also how bloated I feel. I decide I should eat even less since I can't be active feeling like this. My mother, aunt and children visit. I feel privileged to have so much love. The nurse tells me I will have the stress and stomach tests tomorrow. She explains that the esophagus test is not very pleasant. This has been the story of my life lately—pain, tests and more pain and discomfort. I find that the nurses do not like to be disturbed too much. I'm not far from the unit desk and I hear them talking about their outings, families, etc. If they do come in, it is only to attend to your request and never any longer. Florence Nightingale has long gone with her words of comfort and her patience. I do have to say I have met a few nurses who have chosen the right profession.

My legs are so sore I have trouble walking to the elevator and back. Ken had stopped at the general practitioner's office to pick up my file in hopes it might give insight to the doctors. I decided to call my employer and tell them what was currently happening. How I miss home! I pray and ask God why he is doing this, what is his reason?

January 13, 1987

I could not sleep for the pain and anxiety. I was not given breakfast because of the tests scheduled that day and I feel very weak. I took a shower and thought, "Could I be diabetic?" Surely, with all the tests they had done, that would have been revealed. Arterial blood test was done during which I fainted again. An ECG was done and I was sent for my esophagus test. It was terrible, the nurse was right. Tubes were put down my throat and, as liquids were put down the tubes were moved. Another test I wouldn't wish on anyone. The heart stress test was rebooked for tomorrow. I felt a bit stronger after some toast. Ken came to visit and friends also came to see me in the afternoon. The doctor came in and said my carbon dioxide was low. "Are they finding out something?" I thought. He continued, "But I'm almost positive you were hyperventilating and that probably has something to do with your fainting." Hyperventilating, why would I hyperventilate in the shower or while sitting and looking at a magazine, etc.? I was then informed a lung scan would be done for possible clots.

January 14, 1987

Again, I could not sleep well because of pain and discomfort. I was given a "Nitro" before the lung scan and the stress test was put on hold because I was too weak. I felt a bit stronger after some soup and spent an hour visiting. My day revolved around visitors. Although I would tire quickly, the visits kept me sane and gave me reason to keep fighting.

January 15, 1987

Last night was terrible with heart palpitations, pain in my arms and chest, numbness and general soreness and discomfort. I was given "Nitro" at 11 p.m. I finally managed to finish the stress test with difficulty. I felt extremely ill all day. I tried to sleep sitting up because of the pain.

January 16, 1987

At 12:30 a.m., I suddenly awoke with very sore and numb arms and legs. I called the nurse and a resident doctor from the next ward was called in. He looked at me and said, "Now relax, we can't do much until morning anyway." I don't know what had caused the head noises that woke me so suddenly, but I was afraid to fall asleep in case it happened again. It is hard to express how frightened and alone I felt. I knew I was talking to the doctor and nurse. Yet I felt far away, like it wasn't me talking to them. My ears were ringing and I was so weak I couldn't move. What was happening? How I wished someone would stay with me for awhile. I looked at the pictures on my nightstand of Ken and the children. I picked up the phone to call Ken but put it down. I had to go through this night on my own. He had to work and I had asked too much of him already. I felt that if I was to live that night I had to keep awake. I kept writing notes to get me through that terrible night. At that time, I made a promise that, if I lived through this, I'd write a book to help others. If I didn't make it, I hope that my children would do it for me. I think of all the people I love and those who love me. I hope that, if I have hurt someone along the way, I would be forgiven. I pray out loud, "Dear God do not forsake me. I love and trust in you. I know you can help me. If it be your wish, please let me live and help me to function so I can once again help and care for those I love."

As I finish my prayer, I look towards the window and although it is the middle of the night the window lights up. Then the light becomes like a large oval picture frame. To the left in the picture I see my father and near and slightly behind him is his mother and father, my dear grandparents. Then I see my close friend who died as a teenager. Then my other grandparents came into this picture. People who had died and I had known, came into the background of the picture. Then it was full and they were all smiling. At first I'm frightened, but I suddenly feel a warmth and peace come over me. I feel good and I don't hurt. I can't believe my body doesn't hurt. I hear myself say out loud, "I can't be with you now, Rachelle is still so young and I am still needed here. Thank you for your love." The picture fades to a light and goes. I am shaken but feel a faith like never before. God was listening. I now had proof. I knew he would help me and had given me strength to go on. I was thankful for the few moments of relief from pain. I made a decision to keep this to myself for now, as no one would believe me, especially as ill as I was. If I had any doubts before about life after death, It was now gone. My belief in God was strongly reaffirmed.

It's 2:30 a.m. and the pain sets in again as strong as ever. I pick up the phone again to call Ken and put it back down. My upper back is so tender I can't lie back on it. I stay sitting up again. I realize that I have been told by God to accept these hard times, but I still wish for some reprieve. I decide to write notes again, but I'm in a daze and my left hand and left side of my face feel numb. I begin to feel unsafe in this hospital. My understanding was that one would get help in these institutions. The nurse stops to peek around the curtain and goes without a word. I think of my home and fall asleep. I dream I'm in my garden, feeling well, and Rachelle and Ken ask me to go biking with them. We are all riding together and the wind is in my face and I'm going faster and faster. I wake up and cry.

When the doctor came in, I knew I was talking to him, but it was like I was in a tunnel. That morning I was scheduled to have a spine x-ray. I blacked out and wondered what caused it. Linda, my good friend, came to visit and Ken came during his lunch hour. I wanted to hold their hands and never let go. I was given Elavil that night to help me sleep.

January 17, 1987

The medication helped me get some sleep, but I was in such pain when I awoke. I was given a "Nitro" at 8 a.m. As it was Saturday, I probably will not see a doctor today.

When Ken and the children walked in, I knew why God had spared me and I once again knew why I had to get better. I wanted so much to see my grandchildren and watch them grow up. I wanted to feel the passion Ken and I had once enjoyed. Everything seemed centered around this sickness and it was so unfair to everyone. Again, I gather strength from this visit and the calls I have received from my sister in Montreal and my brother in Fort McMurray.

I felt worse on Sunday. As a result, my Elavil medication was increased. I was told the head internal medicine specialist would see me on Monday.

January 19, 1987

The doctor came in and spoke to me for a few minutes informing me that I would most likely have an angiogram. A neurologist then came in to talk to me and examine me. A cardiologist resident then came to see me and said the angiogram could be risky. I decided, if the test would give us answers, I would go through anything that might shed light on this nightmare.

On January 20 I had another ECG and a holter tape to monitor my heart was put on at 11 a.m. I had to record everything I did for 24 hours, which was not much in a hospital room.

January 21, 1987

Last night was really bad again! Twice I woke up suddenly with my heart racing and decided I would try earplugs to see if it was reflexes from sound. The resident came by and said a cardiologist would be in to discuss the holter tape results and we would discuss whether I should have the angiogram.

I have pain in my legs and upper arms tonight and a severe headache. I wish by some miracle I would be healed tonight. But it is not to be; my pain seems to increase. I wonder if it's my heart and that's why my whole body hurts. I'm given Adalat for suspected angina or heart muscle spasm. I can't imagine why I'm given medication before a diagnosis, but if it helps I'll take it. By this time I have escaped into my fourth Daniel Steel book. Little does she know how she has helped me through my tears, pain and loneliness.

January 27, 1987

Six days have passed and nothing has changed. What was happening to my life? Where had my sense of humor and stamina gone? How long could I keep this up without breaking at the seams? I couldn't believe it, this was the third year of this hell.

It was decided that an angiogram might give us some answers. The cardiologist intern came in and said, "You might want to reconsider before signing this form. You realize that there have been cases of puncture, heart attack and some mortality rate from angiogram. Think about it now." I was stunned! What was she saying to me? She put the form on the table and left. I had not yet seen a cardiologist and should have insisted on seeing one. I was so scared and confused I didn't know what to do. I prayed for guidance and couldn't get a hold of Ken at the time. I had said I would do anything, hadn't I? I signed the form.

I went for the angiogram at 11:30 a.m. By the time I got up there I was visibly shaking from fright. The cardiologist was far different from the lady resident doctor. He was reassuring and said everything would be fine. Because of my allergy to dyes, I was given Benedryl. The doctor talked to me all the while he was doing the test and kept reassuring me. I was thankful for his reassurance but thought more than once that I couldn't believe I was going through this.

Once the test was completed, I was taken to the recovery room and watched for possible bleeding. I had finally stopped shaking and was relieved I was still alive. The cardiologist came in and said they did not find any blockages. He also said that it was a good idea to have the test because of my symptoms. Whatever I have, it can't be my heart. "Could a virus have affected my heart as well?" I wondered.

January 28, 1987

The head internal specialist came in with a group of interns and said, "We have concluded that the involuntary muscle spasms are due to the lack of carbon dioxide in your blood, thus causing poor circulation to your arms and legs. Nothing extraordinary was found during the tests. I think you should continue on Adalat and have the Nitro handy." He advised me to try exercising. I assured him I would do as much as I possibly could. I then told him that if nothing else could be done, I wished to go home.

As he left, I could hear him laugh and say to the students, "All Mrs. Stremecki probably needs is a good dose of steroids." They laughed and, as I cried, I thought, "How sad someone in his capacity would say something like that to so many future doctors." I vowed to do everything in my power to never go to a hospital again.

As soon as I got home, I purchased tapes and books on positive living and healing and relaxation. I had made an appointment with the dietitian and followed the diet rigidly. By spring 1987, I had the following symptoms:
- Congestion
- Pain in arms and legs
- Pain in the stomach and trouble digesting
- Pulsating and ringing in the left ear

- Involuntary muscle movements in the arms and legs.
- Pressure and pain in the head and neck
- Upper back pain
- Dizziness and vertigo
- Pins and needles feeling in the arms and legs
- Sore joints
- Head noises upon falling asleep
- Weakness and extreme fatigue
- Memory problems
- Eyesight problems (couldn't stand brightness)
- Skin rashes
- Redness and swelling of hands and feet.

Needless to say, at this point nothing had improved! The Adalat did not eliminate most of my problems, but did help the chest discomfort to a certain extent. I decided if I were to survive this, I would have to start researching this myself. I sent for a major medical book, a book on nutrition and an allergy book. I devoured these and, armed with a list, went back to the doctor who had laughed with the students. I mentioned the environmental aspect and also asked about connective tissue disorders. "What about allergies?" I asked him.

He looked at me as if I had completely lost it and said, "Now you have been looked at by many doctors and you have nothing seriously wrong with you. You are really reading into this, and it will get you nowhere reading all those medical books." He said I should keep taking the Adalat, as he was sure it was mostly stress. I assured him that by now I was definitely stressed as well.

On the way home I couldn't speak. I knew what Ken was thinking. This had been another waste of time and energy not to mention Health Care money. I was sure of one thing, I knew I would never go to this doctor again. I made a decision to start with a new general practitioner. Someone who might just have a totally new perspective on this whole thing.

Summer 1987

In the summer of 1987, I met an acquaintance that informed me his daughter had married a general practitioner and that he was well liked. I decided I would call him for an appointment. He was young and might just have new knowledge about certain things.

In July, I arrived at his office. He was nice and asked what he could do for me. I started my story and noticed he seemed a bit overwhelmed. As I continued, he looked at his watch and I felt like I was taking his time unnecessarily. I felt he should know the background if he was to try and help me. He said he would do what he could for me and asked me to go into the other room for an examination. He checked me and booked blood work, a chest x-ray and an appointment with an allergist. The hardest part about seeing a new doctor was going through some of the same tests again, but I was very determined to get answers.

The tests showed nothing significant, only an allergy to dust and mold. The doctor thought this might account for some of the congestion. Another ECG was done and it too showed nothing significant.

A number of appointments were booked for me. One appointment was with an ENT specialist for answers about the fullness in the left ear and side of the face. I had been to this doctor for a tonsillectomy when I was about 33 years old. I was also booked with an older internist who dealt with heart problems. Also, I was booked with a different internal medicine specialist. This general practitioner was really concerned but confused and was also looking for answers.

The new internal medicine specialist seemed to focus on my heart. He did another ECG and had me come back several times. He also discovered I had ulcers and gave me medication for this. He and the general practitioner conferred back and forth. After a few months of appointments, it was suggested I go on tranquilizers. I was told it was most likely "my age" or a nervous condition. They both agreed, however, that a lot of the symptoms did not point to these things.

There were times that summer when I thought, "No one will ever find out what is wrong with me. I will just have to live day by day. Somehow, something or someone seemed to keep saying, "Keep trying."

Fall 1987

In September I decided to try going back to work. My symptoms seemed to lessen a bit over the summer. I loved my work in student evaluation and hoped to one day complete my degree. It felt good to be back amongst my co-workers. As the day went by, I would, at times, be in tears because of the pain in my body. My feet and hands were so sore and swollen. I was determined that this monster would not make me quit work again. A few months after going back to work my symptoms worsened.

Christmas was coming and there was so much to do. The joy of seeing family and friends made it all worthwhile. By January, I had addtional things happening to me. There was a gurgling noise in my chest and I was short of breath. I was sore in the left side of my abdomen. The cramps in my legs and feet were much worse.

February 1988

In February, Ken had the opportunity to work at the Calgary Winter Olympics. Although it was not a good time for me, I felt it was a great opportunity for him to get away from it all. He had been through so much coping with my illness. The month dragged on for me with meetings to firm up negotiations for the construction of our acreage home. We had to pack and move into a rental house and it was very busy at work. I now wonder how I did it. It is amazing how much a body can tolerate.

In March 1988 we moved into a rental house while our acreage house was being built. All the children helped us move. I was exhausted but determined not to let this "condition" run my life. I had to keep alive and sane. The sane part being the most difficult at this time.

The doctor appointments continued and by late spring my neurological symptoms were worse. I would be awakened by head noises. It was like someone took hold of my brain and shook it. It made me totally dizzy and it was terrifying. I would break into a sweat and often felt like fainting, especially towards morning. The muscle and bone aches were incredible. I was more congested and the leg cramps were more frequent.

As summer progressed, our acreage house was coming along nicely. It was a white cape cod, our dream home! How many times I looked at the partly finished house and wondered if I ever would be well enough to live in it. We encountered the usual problems with building a home, but managed to cope with it all.

Ken started fencing as soon as possible. The sooner we could bring our horse home, the sooner we would eliminate boarding costs. I recall trying to paint the fence and crying with pain as my hand cramped around the paintbrush. I refused to let this illness stop me from taking part in all of this. God, where was the person I was supposed to be?

Doctor appointments and tests still took a great portion of our time. The social functions were very few. How grateful I am for the love of my family and friends. They stood by us when socializing could not be a priority.

I devoured books and articles to try and find answers. I came upon a disease called lupus, a disease in which the immune systems attacks the good cells. I wrote this down to mention it to my general practitioner during my next visit. By this time, I think he was ready to give up on me and about as discouraged as I was. The house building took 2 months longer than expected.

Robert and Lorena were expecting their first child—our first grandchild, I could hardly wait! On September 4, 1988, Daniel was born. He was perfect and healthy. God had given us a great gift. I couldn't get enough of him when I first saw him. How we cherished these good times, which helped us through the bad ones.

In October 1988 we moved into our new home. I focused on the positive; otherwise, I couldn't have done what I did with the pain I had. At times I could barely walk because my feet were so swollen. I can't begin to try and share with you how tired I was. I had so many projects I wanted to do in our new home, like sewing curtains, putting up pictures, making cushions, etc. I had always loved decorating our home and this one would be such fun to do. I was so ill that the project waited and waited.

Christmas 1988 was nice out in the country. Having a grandchild made it so very special. Again most of my family was able to make it that year. Ken and the children helped with the meal and cleaned up. As I sat in the living room in the still of the night, I thanked God for yet another Christmas. Surely if this kept up I would not see many more. I had contacted a lupus specialist in Calgary and was waiting for his call.

December 29, 1988 (notes from diary)

The pain seems worse than ever. I am so congested and can't sleep. As I sit in our living room and write this, I think of silly things like ending this pain. It is a morbid thought because I don't think I could do it. I love my family and have so much to live for. I cannot share this deep, dark depressive time in its entirety with family and friends. I know they have heard enough and preferred not to hear much more. I have slept only a few hours because of the pain and discomfort. "Please God, I beg you to help me. Why are you letting this happen to me? What do you want of me?" It is now 4 years and I have such trouble handling this at times. I'm so discouraged.

Our anniversary is here and I so desperately want Ken to have the woman he married. Rachelle is only 14 years old and I want so much to see her grow up. I have to keep trying! I've just found out that the lupus specialist does not think it is lupus. That is good news, but then what is it? Why then are my legs cramping and I'm so puffy and sore? My left ear is ringing and pulsating and my left side is so sore. I swear again that if I ever get even a bit more energy, I will write about this. How I love my new grandson and want to see him grow up. I will see him grow up!

January 1989

What would this year bring? At this point I felt it could not get much worse, it had to improve. I kept telling my internal specialist that I had incredible pain in my lower left side. I also asked for another neurological opinion.

By the month of March, I had been back to this specialist a number of times. On March 6, 1989, he said, "Annette, I feel this is not life threatening as you have been seen by a lot of doctors." He felt that I should accept it and try to live with it. I could tell this specialist was as bewildered as was my general practitioner. He ordered more blood work and a urine test. When I asked him about the neurologist, he said, "Maybe your general practitioner can do that." "I'm so confused and annoyed that no one can help me. Five years ago I could dance, bike, play tennis, etc. I now have trouble walking and in addition to all these symptoms, I have this gurgling and severe pain in my left side," I said. He looked at me and I knew we had come to a standstill and that he was no longer sympathetic to my condition. His parting statement was, "You know, you may want to consider taking dancing lessons. It would only hurt a little and everything might go away." I was stunned and said, "Thank you doctor," as I walked out.

As I drove home I could barely see for the tears. What was wrong with me, did I not say I would keep at this until I got answers? Nevertheless, I decided this internal specialist might see other patients, but certainly not me.

The next day I kept the appointment with my gynecologist of 20 years. He had successfully brought Rachelle into the world after a hard pregnancy and difficult delivery. I explained my dilemma. He said he felt I had neurological symptoms and should have been referred to another neurologist. He asked again if I had been given tests for MS. I told him I had and he indicated if my general practitioner would not give me a referral to get back to him. He checked my ovaries and said everything seemed fine. His words of support and encouragement helped.

That week I went back to see my general practitioner. He examined me again and said he suspected an ovarian cyst. I was booked with another doctor for an ultrasound and a barium x-ray. I began to feel like a frightened child who wants to hide or run away from a frightening situation. I was developing a phobia towards doctors and anything to do with medicine. However, I also knew that was probably the only way I would get answers and hopefully some help.

I dug out my positive thinking books and worked at it again. I knew I was at a point were I had to help myself somehow. At this point, I also felt that out of the 30-some doctors I had seen, quite a few must be as frustrated as I was. My general practitioner was up front with me and said, "We'll see what this doctor says and, to tell you the truth, I don't know what else I can do for you."

At the end of March I received the results from my tests. The ultrasound showed a fluid mass on the left side of my abdomen. The colon was okay; except for a polyp that he felt should not be removed at this time. I was to book another appointment with my gynecologist to follow up on the report that would be sent to him.

That same week I had an appointment with another neurologist who seemed like a nice, older gentleman. He listened to my story and said he felt it was vestibular neuritis since Meniere's disease had been eliminated. He seemed more concerned about the dizziness than anything else. From my understanding of the brief explanation, it was an inflammation of the inner ear or something of that nature. He prescribed Gravol for this. I tried taking these but felt worse in the morning and it gave me diarrhea.

Through all of this I missed as little work as I could. My position with the school district was important to me. At this time I was inundated with work and added responsibilities. For a number of years I had been asking for a reclassification, which would incorporate all I was doing. Unable to continue my course work towards my degree, I was doing consulting work on a clerk's salary. I stayed on because I loved my work. The in-services and individual contacts with school personnel were stimulating and educational. As with most major organizations, it was political and advancement often depended on whom you knew and how close one could get to this one or that one. After being a partner in a private business where recognition for a job well done was important, working for a major organization was an eye opener. I will always be grateful to those colleagues who supported and encouraged me.

One morning the head secretary called me and said, "Annette, there is an envelope here, which I think belongs to you. I opened it in error." On this envelope was my general practitioner's name, which was misspelled, and my office address rather than his. It was from the Humanity Hospital. The reason she had opened it was because the assistant superintendent's name was very similar. What an error the hospital had made.

At lunch I started to read and now understood how a patient is looked at and can be misunderstood. As I read, I couldn't believe my eyes. It was so full of exaggerations in regards to what I had said. The first neurologist stated that I thought I had a brain tumor because there was family history of these. The truth being, I was asked what my family history was and I had mentioned this. On and on it went. Some were actual lies about certain things. As previously mentioned, it read that I had left the hospital after a CAT scan without permission. I couldn't believe this. I had asked the nurse to see if I could leave and she returned saying I could. Another stated I had been discharged from the hospital in good condition after eliminating Meniere's disease in January 1986. I left in a wheelchair with all sorts of problems.

By the time I was half way through the reports I was in tears. So this is the kind of thing that went from doctor to doctor. This was the respect a patient got as a human being. Everything was written in a way that the medical profession looked good and that I was a crazy middle-aged woman. As I kept reading, I now understood why I was being treated like a hypochondriac. There it was in plain writing. The psychiatrist from the Hope Clinic had stated "possible hypochondria" in his report. Things were now becoming clearer. If such an institution would even give the slightest hint of such a diagnosis, why not believe it. It made things much simpler for the medical doctors. I closed my office door and cried. Somehow God had permitted this error so I would be aware of what was happening and why some doctors were treating me in the way they were. How could anyone possibly think I was "faking" it? It was mind-boggling how they could ever think a patient liked to go through all the horribly painful tests I had been through. Did they actually believe we wanted to spend our precious time focusing on this nightmare of an illness?

Apart from all the lies, the test results were interesting. I read things that had never been shared with us. In some cases they were stated as borderline but had never been followed up. I found out I had generalized osteoarthritis in my spine that had not been discussed with me. This I figured probably accounted for the back pain I had. As I went over these, I wondered if the doctors even went over these before seeing a patient. "Most likely not," I thought.

The afternoon went by slowly, I was totally distracted by what I had just read. I was mad, very mad. This was not characteristic of me. I always was giving people the benefit of the doubt. I swore I would do something about this! How many other people were being treated in this manner.

What a letdown to think people I held in high esteem could be so unjust and unreliable.

Driving home at the end of the day was difficult for me due to the light-headedness, dizziness and the pain. This night, however, the tears made it hard to see. I had been working so hard at being positive and here I was stressed to the hilt again by what I had read. I shared this with Ken and he tried his best to calm me down. He was furious that this error could have occurred in the first place. Once he had read it, he agreed the reports were most disturbing.

The next day I called the supervisor of records at the Humanity Hospital and explained the error while elaborating on the graveness of such an error. She was apologetic and said she would look into the matter and send another copy of the records to my general practitioner. At this point I didn't think I wanted him to have a copy but he had requested them. Fair enough, I would be ready for his reaction once he had received these. The statement from the little "hawk" psychiatrist was now having a snowball effect. The only thing that this snowball could do is squash me at the bottom of the hill.

This episode left me devastated for quite some time, although now I was aware of a lot. Rather than look at the negative aspect I began to look at it as a blessing that would enable me to be on the lookout with people in the medical community. To hell with the darn reports, I would keep looking for help. Every time I was at my lowest, I felt that someone picked me up and told me not to give up.

April 7, 1989

I will again see my general practitioner. So far he has been the most supportive, although he is confused that he can't find any answers. He agrees my gynecologist should see me again to discuss the test findings. He suggested I take coated Aspirin for the muscle and joint pain.

April 11, 1989

Today I have my appointment with my gynecologist and he apologizes for not having noticed the problem found during the ultrasound. He wants to do a laparoscopy and I agree as my left side is very sore and hurts whenever I walk. As I drive home, I wonder if maybe this might be the cause of most of my problems.

April 23, 1989

I check into the Humanity Hospital for the laparoscopy. The place I vowed I would never come to again. At least, this time it is for a purpose—to determine what exactly was seen on the ultrasound. Ken and I are confident, maybe, just maybe, this will give us answers and things could get back to normal.

The usual routine happens. I'm given blood tests and an intern checks me over and asks the same questions I've answered so many times already. At approximately 12:30 a.m. I asked the student nurse for Tylenol for pain. She came back with two Tylenol with Codeine. I told her my chart indicated I had a severe allergy to morphine. "Was Codeine not in the same family?" I informed her I had a severe reaction from Codeine in the past. She assured me it was not in the morphine family and would work much better than plain Tylenol. I closed my eyes and waited for the Tylenol to take effect.

About ½ hour later I had trouble breathing. I felt like a brick had fallen on my chest. I rang the nurse buzzer and a student nurse came in. She called the head nurse who immediately took my blood pressure. She then called the intern on call. I could hear them talking but it was as if they were so far away. I heard one say, "her blood pressure is dropping rapidly, call in the team." I begged them to help me! My thoughts were of Ken and the children and I heard myself praying out loud, "God help me, please help me." The heart team started an I.V. and medication was administered. I was also given Nitroglycerin. "She's pulling out of it, her blood pressure is back up," I heard someone say. My chest was starting to feel better but I felt so very weak. I was given an oxygen mask. The nurses came in regularly and checked my blood pressure during the night

In the morning another young resident intern came in to see me. She sat by my bedside looking very indifferent and said, "I've taken the time to read all your reports and that certainly tells me a lot doesn't it?" She grabbed the oxygen mask and yanked it off. "How could you do such a thing, we have to look after real patients and have no time for this," she said. The nurse in the corner looked pale as she watched and said, "But doctor, this patient's blood pressure dropped rapidly; she definitely had some sort of severe reaction." It is hard to express how I felt when I heard this. Disbelief would first begin to explain it. She had seen the very reports I had recently received in error. It had to be a reaction to the "hawk" psychiatrist indicating I could be a probable hypochondriac. This nightmare would never end! It seemed like a movie that was happening to someone else, not me. By that one statement, that doctor had made me a prisoner unable to escape. How ironical that my focus at work was to ensure that students were not falsely labeled and would be given the opportunity to live up to their potential. Now, it was I who had been falsely labeled. I lay there frightened and sick to my stomach but could not vomit. I thought of suing the doctor who was responsible for this. We all know for a fact that the medical profession sticks together like glue and the stress of such action would be too much to take. We would probably lose and we couldn't afford it anyway.

April 24, 1989

My gynecologist came in and we discussed what had happened. I explained that I had pain in my left arm and dull pain in the center of the chest. I also had a gurgling sensation when I took a deep breath. He said the laparoscopy would have to be rebooked and he would ask a cardiologist to come and look at me. I can't believe this has happened and I have to come back to this place again and that I took time off to have this happen to me.

That evening Ken and Rachelle came to see me. I feel bad they have to come to a hospital again, but seeing them is like a ray of sunshine. They cannot believe what has happened and that I have to have the procedure rebooked.

The cardiologist who was supposed to see me had just left for Germany. Another cardiologist, who had recently operated on my gynecologist, was then asked to see me. On the morning of April 25 a third one came as the second one could not make it either. He listened to my heart and said it was fine to go home but the laparoscopy would have to be rebooked, as it was safer not to put me to sleep now. Before I left, my gynecologist said, "We'll book the laparoscopy and the surgery all at once since we know there is a cyst in there." This would be booked in about 2 weeks. As I dressed, I shed more tears and wondered how long a human being could take all of this. At this time, my total symptoms were the following:

- Fatigue, weakness and fainting spells
- Pulsating and ringing in the left ear
- Pain in neck, shoulder and arms especially the left one.
- Sore left side of abdomen
- Crinkling feeling in the left side of the chest
- Sore muscles and joints
- Sore calves
- Hands and feet either white or red, swollen and burning.
- Swelling of the left leg and foot
- Shaky
- Severe upper back pain
- Numbness especially in the left hand and left side of face.
- Weight gain
- Memory problems, word recognition and usage and spelling of certain words.

The following are findings that I was aware of at this time. Most of these through the medical reports I had received in error. Others were suspected by doctors and discussed with me:

- Vestibular neuritis
- Hiatus Hernia
- Esophageal motility disturbances
- Osteoarthritis in spine
- Dominant right coronary circulation
- Right ventricle prominent and short left Mainstem Coronary Artery.
- Growth in left side of abdomen.

The findings were apparently not significant enough to follow-up, except for the growth in the ovary area.

It is unfortunate that so many medical professionals are so detached from the human aspect. I'm not generalizing when I say this. I have come across and still see some great doctors who remember that patients are someone's mother, father, daughter, son, wife, husband or grandparent. They respect our input and take time to listen to their patients. To all you great doctors, I take this time to send you a bouquet for the person you are. Caring for people should be a compassionate exchange between patient and doctor.

May 14, 1989

It's Mother's Day and I have to book into the hospital again. As we approach, I feel nauseous and wonder if I should cancel the whole thing and go home. After the last few visits, I'm definitely not comfortable booking in again. I have armed myself with a list of opium derivatives to prevent an allergic fiasco like the last time.

Once I'm in my room I go through the same routine again. I wonder why all my history has to be taken again and by now I'm reluctant to say anything. I'm informed that I'll be going up to the operating room on Monday at 1:30 p.m. I try to read but am too nervous and can't concentrate. My mind wonders to our home, my family and to positive thoughts. How I'm envious of people now able to work in their gardens. It's spring and here I am stuck in the hospital again. "Quit feeling sorry for yourself, there are many more people worse off than you," I say to myself. God will surely take care of me. I decide to do positive imagery. I'm in a field walking towards a stream. Everything is green and the sky is blue. I see animals grazing in a meadow and wild flowers all around me in bright and warm colors. As I walk, I pray and talk to my Dad in heaven. Now my family and friends surround me. We're picnicking and laughing and talking. I feel good and start to run in the field and feel the warm wind on my face. I run and run without pain. A nurse walks in and I'm brought back to reality. "Yes, this operation must make a difference to the way I feel." I have to stay positive.

In the evening Rachelle, Ken, Joanne, Dennis, Robert, Lorena and my darling little Daniel came to visit. They spoil me, as usual, with gifts and plants. It is their visit, however, that is the greatest gift of all. At 8:30 p.m. I was given an enema. What an "ending" for Mother's Day!

I didn't sleep very well, but was not about to ask for anything to help me sleep. I had a shower and the nurse then put in the I.V. The doctor came in to reassure me and tell me it was sometimes difficult to remove a fluid-type cyst. Also, that he would not do the laparoscopy because we knew that there was a cyst and did not see a need to investigate further. He explained that I would go up to the operating room later as another patient of his had come in during the night and he would do her surgery first. The extra wait did not help my nerves but I felt that if the other patient needed it first, then I could wait a while longer.

Ken said he would be here when I woke up. I would of felt so alone without his support and love. I thanked God for him, my family and friends. I asked God to be with me and help the doctor with the surgery.

On the way to the operating room I thought of how many times I had been put to sleep and how it still frightened me. The doctor was reassuring and I felt in good hands. He recently had heart surgery and said, "Annette, I now know what it's like to be the patient and it has made me look at things differently." I had always thought of him as a caring and dedicated doctor. Thanks to his help, we have Rachelle, a child I thought we would lose.

I opened my eyes and saw Ken. Still groggy, I can't believe it's over. The assisting doctor explains to us that they had removed a fluid-type mass the size of a large grapefruit. My gynecologist then agrees we should dangle it in front of a few doctors' noses. No wonder my side hurt so much! The surgery left me sleepy and congested. The nurse came in and sat me in a chair for a while. I remembered the feeling well from previous surgery, like your gut is about to spill out!

On the third day I was started on fluids, but still had the I.V. I noticed that the muscle pain was not so bad. "Was I allergic to some foods?" I wondered. Maybe it was the removal of such a large cyst that made my joints and muscles feel a bit better. My catheter and drain tubes were removed the following day. I decided to walk to the pantry to get some juice.

A group of nurses came in at shift-change and a stern-looking nurse said very loudly, "Well, do we need an enema or did you finally have a bowel movement?" If she would have said it louder, the next room would have heard it and maybe they did. The other nurses just grinned and looked at each other. This could have been done a little more discretely at another time or in a lower voice. I realized the importance of the question but please a little respect. As I looked at her, I thought it didn't look like she had had a bowel movement for a number of months. I still had not lost my sense of humor totally! My temperature was taken and I was told I had a low-grade temperature. This was nothing new for me as I had been told this a number of times. A blood test followed to check for infection.

My doctor came in for his rounds and said I could go home on Sunday. I was now on solid foods and I had the I.V. taken out. It felt so good to be rid of all the tubes. My arms and legs were not so painful and I was so grateful for this. Maybe this was the beginning of better times at last. I still had a number of the other symptoms but I couldn't expect to be rid of everything in a few days and how nice to be rid of the pain in my left side when I walk. My incision is starting to heal and I'm happy to see this, as I'm not usually a good healer.

My neighbor in my room is a nice young Spanish lady. We talk and I discover she is the patient the doctor had to operate on before me. We had some good visits and short walks together. Ken and the children, family and friends were often here to visit. My godchild was here to see me and it meant so much to me that she would take time from her busy schedule as a teacher. As I write this, I cry because we have just found out that she recently passed away at such a young age. I know God loves her and has her in his care.

I think of all the people who have to spend their life in a hospital setting and wonder how they cope with it. How did my Dad handle those many years in a nursing home, incapacitated? I remember coming to visit him and finding a staff member shoving food down his throat with a soup-spoon. He was gagging and she was saying, "Come on, eat your food, hurry up." How could she do this to my poor Dad who in his whole life would not hurt anyone? I yelled at her and pushed her away telling her that if she ever came close to my Dad again, I would sit on her and shove food down her throat at the same rate. We reported this employee and she was dismissed. How many elderly and ill people are treated this way? Many, so where is the proper supervision of these people? This illness is teaching me how important support and love is, especially at these times.

May 19, 1989

I woke up not feeling very well this morning. I had the same zinging noise in my head I had previously experienced and it woke me up often. Was it something I ate now that I was off the I.V.? I had a shower and felt very weak, like I was about to faint. I drank some juice and had some porridge and felt a bit better. I decided if I went to the beauty parlor, it might improve my disposition. I was very tired when I came back and concluded I was not as strong as I thought I was.

That day was filled with visitors. Some of my co-workers came and we had some good laughs. My mother and her friend came, as well as the children. Our good friends Linda and John also were up for a visit bearing gifts as well. In the evening another group from work was in to visit. I called Ken and Rachelle before going to sleep. I was exhausted from all the company, but the day had gone by fast for a change. I dreamt of Ken and that we are both happy and well. "A dream," I thought when I woke up, "it was only a dream."

The following day my gynecologist and I had a good talk. He talked about his pending retirement next month and I assured him he would be missed. I was very congested that day and thought it might be from something I ate. I looked at my garden books, watched the news and tried to avoid the "dragon lady" nurse who was on duty. I wondered again how these institutions screened their staff and how these people could continue working at a job they obviously disliked. Rachelle and Ken came over after supper and we watched North and South together.

May 21, 1989

I awoke feeling a profound joy at the thought of going home. I was fortunate that someone had taken the time to give me communion and pray with me. As I prayed, I felt a feeling of peace and love, knowing God was with me.

My tummy was itchy from the tape over my incision so I asked the nurse for some cream for the rash. It was the same nurse so I hesitated to ask her. She returned and said, "Try this, we'll bring you everything on the cart before calling your doctor you know." Why would she comment like that? Why would she think I would ask for the doctor about a tape rash? Things started to get a little clearer now. This was the same hospital that had the report from the dear little psychiatrist, she must have read it or been told by someone. She had not said that to be humorous. It saddened me to see how cruel people can be. Just then, Ken and Rachelle came around the corner and he said, "Are you ready?" It felt so great to leave! I couldn't wait to step into our house. When I did, it felt so big and sunny and our golden retriever Tara was there to greet me. If felt so good to be home!

June 14, 1989

I went to see the gynecologist for a postoperative visit. He assumed my ovaries had not been functioning for years. As he was retiring, he suggested my general practitioner start me on estrogen therapy. I wondered why I had never been given a hormone test earlier in view of all the problems I had been having. Could this also be a part of my problems? I knew that hormonal imbalance could have serious consequences. I was back at work by June 19, with hopes that things would improve further because of the surgery.

July 1989

My hopes were crushed. By mid July all the symptoms were back, except the pain that I had experienced on the left side of my abdomen. Added to the others was a new one, which was electric-shock-like feelings going through my body at different times and places. Had I exhausted medical assistance? I thought of curling up on my bed and giving up. I knew better, I would keep going.

At the end of July I went to see my general practitioner again. He said, "This is incredible, it has to be some form of systemic disorder." He ordered blood work for a hormonal count. My estrogen level was very low. I was started on estrogen patch therapy and calcium. After 2 weeks the hot flushes and night sweats were not so frequent. I was thankful for any of the symptoms that could be eliminated. After a month I knew I was dealing with more than one thing because the other symptoms continued.

In mid August I wrote to the director of the Hope Clinic to share with him what had previously happened at this clinic and what was happening since then. I told him I was anxious for feedback and possible direction from him. I never did get an answer. This confirms how important the patient is.

My position with the school district was 10-month and part-time. I could no longer work full time. I returned in September ready for the challenges that always presented themselves and anxious to see everyone. At this time I was starting to have problems with my vision, such as spots and blurriness. I seemed to get even more tired towards the end of the day and my calves would hurt so much I would cry.

I felt at this point that I could no longer share with family and friends. I knew they had trouble listening to this on an ongoing basis and feel helpless. I continued to write in my diary and it has become a friend to me. I had to take things day by day. I had this incredible need to get better and was determined to keep looking for help. Obviously, this is a chronic illness of some sort, but what? I wondered again about lupus and decided to call the specialist in Calgary. It was a sunny day and I prayed that God would send me his light and guide me in the right direction and to the right people. I come so close to giving up, it frightens me.

November 1989

November is here and I'm still dealing with the same symptoms. About a week ago I had a severe seizure-like experience. I don't know what else to call it. I awoke with a terrible zinging sensation in my head, but this time it was like a shock going through my arms and legs. God, this monster in my body is frightening! I have to stop sharing everything with Ken, as he is affected by all of this and I'm afraid he might get ill also. I sometimes wake him up if I scream during the night, but I often stay in the living room most of the night because the pain keeps me awake.

We were invited to Montreal for my niece's wedding. We decided that we would go despite the way I felt. Maybe the trip would do us both good. Financially it was not a good idea, but it might provide an opportunity to see a doctor in Montreal. I asked my sister to make an appointment at the clinic she had been going to. An appointment was scheduled for January 3, 1990.

During December all my symptoms persisted. I also had the flu that left me even more congested. The pain in the left side of my neck, left arm and chest pain persisted. I decided I should maybe stop writing in my diary; maybe I was dwelling too much on it by doing this. This was easier said than done because writing kept me sane.

Our trip to Montreal was nice, as far as being with family. My appointment at the clinic was disappointing. No one saw me, except for a nurse who photocopied my test results. I was told that the doctor would probably look at them and compare them to my sister Terry's test results to see if there was a similarity. I suppose I was hoping for some sort of miracle and that maybe I'd get some answers. The day after the wedding Ken got a bad flu and Terry and I spent New Years Eve in emergency with him. He was so ill and had to stay in bed that we decided to go to a hotel for the rest of our visit. I was extremely tired and sore. Here we were miles from home and both sick in a hotel. We wondered if we would ever have a good holiday again.

I returned to work part-time in January. I was now wondering how I ever coped. I found it was a necessity to keep as busy as possible so I would not go mad. Daylight breaking was a sight I often witnessed. I felt so bad laying down that I often tried to sleep sitting up in the living room. I was taking Aspirin and because it seemed to help the inflammation I was increasing the dosage too much and my stomach got so sore. As I look at the original notes in my diary they are filled with things like, "What have I got? I can't take this any longer. Please God, help me."

At the end of January 1990 my general practitioner sent me for an ultrasound of the kidneys as the pain in my left side below my rib cage was worse. I decide to cut out all sugars. I have to try things on my own. Also, I decide to eat more vegetables, which seems to help my joints and muscles to some extent. Work is very busy and I'm trying to do full time work on a part-time basis. The famous reclassification is still ongoing regarding all the additional responsibilities I've accumulated during the last 5 years.

On February 8, 1990, I went to see my doctor and was informed that the ultrasound did not show any problems with the kidneys. I told him I still had a lot of pain in my left side and was told to take Aspirin for it.

February 11, 1990

I attended mass with Ken and Rachelle as often as I could. My relationship with God was "topsy-turvy." I questioned him a lot these days. I knew there had to be a reason for what was happening, I just wanted to know why and what was happening. Coming home from mass in a terrible storm, I had an incredible pain in my left side that made me scream. As my pain tolerance was high, I could not believe what was happening. Poor Ken and Rachelle. They were so worried and I felt so bad for them. The storm was getting worse, so Ken decided to drive and meet the ambulance in Sherwood Park rather than trying to drive to the hospital. These severe pains kept coming about 10 minutes apart then would subside a bit. It was like someone was inside me twisting my bowels. Ken and Rachelle followed the ambulance in the storm. I couldn't believe this was happening again. It was like a never-ending nightmare! It had not been a year since my operation, how could I be back in a hospital? "Keep calm, don't lose it or they will really think your nuts," I told myself. It felt like the body I was in wasn't mine. It was totally incomprehensible. I was again given blood work, x-rays and a urine test. I must be radioactive by now I think. The emergency doctor said he could not see anything significant on the x-ray but felt it must be gas pain. Gas pain, did he think that at my age I had never had gas pain! This was no gas pain I told him. "Was it a twisted bowel?" I asked. He didn't think so. I was given a laxative and left with a very sore side while apologizing to Ken and Rachelle. What else could I say? At that moment I wished I would go to sleep and never wake up.

February 14, 1990

Valentines' Day! Another day that reminds me why I have to make it through the rough times. All the children will be over on Sunday and I can't wait to see them. I'm still having pulsating pain on the left side below my rib cage. At the end of February my sister called from Montreal and asked if I had seen the article on chronic fatigue in the Woman's Day magazine. I told her I had read it and was going to bring it to my doctor. Some of the symptoms described were the same as mine. Terry was not well herself and had been under the care of doctors also. I wondered if this was genetic.

March 1990

When I went to see my general practitioner I showed him the article on chronic fatigue syndrome. He glanced at the title quickly and said, "This is very hard to diagnose and very little is known about it." He handed it back to me saying he had already read it. I wondered why doctors felt threatened when we questioned them or informed them of something. Why could they not work with us? He dictated a letter to the gastroenterologist regarding the pain in my left side. An appointment was booked for March 26. Again, I shared with him how very tired I am and how the ringing and pulsating in my left ear is much worse. I also tell him that the joint and muscle pains have come back with a vengeance. I'm reminded not to "dwell on this."

I decided to join our church choir. I miss singing so much and think that possibly it will be good for me. I attended a sing-and-praise day and did not think I would make it through the day because I was in such pain and discomfort. I was proud when I left because I had managed to stay for the day. I'm noticing my recall seems to be getting worse. This really scares me!

This is an especially hard time as a co-worker with the school system passed away from an aneurysm. She was not yet 50 and was awaiting her first grandchild. She had complained of a sore neck and was treated for arthritis and stress. I'm not sure how long she had been complaining of this. We are constantly reminded about seeing a doctor or go to a hospital at the first signs of a heart attack or stroke, yet repeatedly people are sent back home without proper treatment. We would be astounded as to how many people, after informing a doctor of the symptoms, have been sent home and then have a heart attack or a stroke.

My former brother-in-law has recently passed away of a heart attack. His family had brought him to the hospital (in which there is a well known heart centre) and he was sent home with a prescription for the flu, only to die a week later. He was a young man. Medical schools must teach their students the art of listening to their patients to attain improved health care.

I continued to keep as busy as possible in an attempt not to dwell on what was ravaging my body. I watched the sunsets, thanked God for another day and asked him to help me cope with the next day. In late March we decided to go to Calgary with some friends for the weekend. I could not refuse Ken after all the time he gave caring for and supporting me. It was a challenge to accept but we were close to John and Linda who had continued to be friends with us through it all. Our husbands went skiing and we decided to do a little shopping and looking around downtown. I quickly tired and prayed that I would last the afternoon without telling Linda how sore and tired I was. I was determined not to spoil her day. When I got back to our room, I cried and swore I would beat this and one day will be able to do "normal" things again. I couldn't even spend a few hours in a store with a friend and didn't know why. I knew in my heart it would kill me, if I gave up.

I kept writing in my diary, although it seemed repetitious. It was like pouring my heart out to someone. Again, I was desperately trying to hide my suffering and frustration. I could see that everyone was fed up with the situation. Obviously friends and family were still there for me, but I could no longer see how they could be. There were times when I would get to an all time low and think of suicide. God, to be rid of all of this at times seemed so good! It was against my beliefs, but I could sympathize with others who had chosen that path.

My Dad, who was a most wonderful man, suffered for years before dying and yet never complained. He used to say, "God loves all those who suffer." He then smiled and added, "Maybe he could love me a little less these days." With my days filled with pain, I would ask him to give me strength and show me how to cope without getting so discouraged. No doubt he has a "top notch" place in heaven.

March 26, 1990

The gastroenterologist that I was referred to was curt. She would ask questions and would not let me finish before interrupting. "Nothing different here," I thought. She said, "I see from your doctor's letter that you have been seeing Drs. so and so, has lupus been diagnosed yet?" I said it had not yet been diagnosed as lupus. "The death rate is high from lupus, you wouldn't want to have that," she continued. I was so flabbergasted at her statement that I could not respond. As she began to walk away, she said, "Please see the receptionist, we will book you for a colonoscopy and put you on Bentylol for muscle spasm." I waited, as I thought she had just gone to speak to the receptionist, but then gathered that we were finished. Another doctor who lacked communication skills, but if she knew what she was doing that's all I cared about. The receptionist booked me for May 17 and gave me some instructions. Another test! I'm in tears as I get into the car. I hate this! Oh how I hate it and want it to end. I tell myself I can't let anyone see me like this and talk myself into accepting this in the hopes it might shed some light on things. It is all part of a storm before a rainbow, I tell myself.

April 7, 1990 (notes from diary)

I'm alone at home and I'm scared. I feel weak, like I'm going to faint. My throat burns and hurts on either side and I have such a bad taste in my mouth. My chest hurts and my heart is pounding. There are pulsating and swishing noises in my ears and head. God, get me through this day. It's Palm Sunday tomorrow and I want to go to church. I'm so tired I have to lie down.

I was determined to sing with the choir on Palm Sunday. I had missed numerous rehearsals but was confident I knew enough to sing with them. I stood with the others and during the second song I became very warm and had to sit down. Someone helped me outside because I felt like I was going to faint. Ken and Rachelle came to me and we went home. So much for that try! I felt terrible. The feelings of guilt were constantly there. We went to Robert's and Lorena's in the afternoon, but I did not feel well. I was not going to let Ken and Rachelle miss this. Being with my children and grandchild was like a tonic for me. It still is and always will be. Their love is the greatest of gifts.

The next day I was unable to work. I could not stay up more than 10 to 15 minutes at a time. I saw another doctor that day, as mine was away. He took a blood test and it indicated I had a high lymph count that he explained indicated a viral infection. Did I have a strange virus ravaging my body? On Tuesday I had to stay home. I was able to sit and listen to Rachelle play the piano. We had a long talk afterwards. These are treasured times. How lucky we are to have such talented and intelligent children. All are musical!

I'm not a good patient and I worry about deadlines at work. On Wednesday I decided I had to go to work. I no sooner got there that I felt like fainting. Joan, a friend and co-worker, took me to my mother's, which was a few blocks away, until Ken could pick me up. How would I ever finish my goals that were to revise a testing manual and other supportive information for the teachers? As well, there were in-services to be prepared and given. I loved my work and hated my body for preventing me from doing the things I loved. I would look at the University calendar and wish I could continue my studies. There were so very many things I could no longer do—like biking, dancing, gardening and racket sports. Even a simple thing like going for a walk was impossible most of the time. I was so mad. What the hell was happening to me? I wanted answers!

Ken, Rachelle and I decided we would make Easter supper. As I looked at them all around the table, I felt warmth in my heart. How I loved them all! I silently thanked God for letting me be there with them. With everyone's help, the day was great. We had some good laughs and laughing is still one of the best medicines.

Every time I did something extra, I paid for it. The next day I was very ill. My left ear and whole left side were terrible. My general practitioner had an ECG done and said everything was okay. He seemed concerned and asked about my work. He suggested I take 2 weeks off. I told him I would consider a week and then we could discuss if I should take more. He reminded me I must be overdoing things and I was stressed because of it. I refrained from telling him that if I could get relief from whatever I had, then I wouldn't be so stressed. It was my medical situation that was so stressful. I hated missing work, I would get so far behind and that wouldn't help matters.

On the way home I thought of the x-rays a dentist had taken and how he had commented that I might have a cyst under a tooth. This was the same dentist who had recently done a root canal and to whom I had said it just didn't feel right. I went to my regular dentist and had other x-rays done, but he said everything seemed okay. This tooth problem was also on the left side, the side of the head that gave me so much trouble. If it continued to bother me, I would get another opinion.

April 24, 1990

I decided to try going back to work. I was behind in everything and I felt I had to try. It was even difficult to dress, as I felt so weak. I drove to the corner of the acreage and stopped for the lights. As I looked up, I experienced pain in my left arm and shoulder. The left side of my face felt numb and the next thing I knew my head was on the steering wheel. I don't remember putting it there, I must have blacked out. I was so very weak and thanked God I hadn't yet gone on the freeway. I got back home and called Lois, my neighbor. I then called my general practitioner and I was told to go to emergency at the Sisters of Charity Hospital. This was a different hospital than the one where I had my surgery. Lois stayed with me until noon. Finally, I was given blood work, x-rays and an ECG. I was told that everything was within the normal range. God, why had this happened to me? Why can't they find out what is wrong and help me? My doctor informed the hospital he would continue to treat me as an outpatient.

The next day was Secretaries' Day and I so wanted to join in with the others, but I could barely make it to my bathroom that morning. My diary that day reads, "Damn, damn, damn, I'm fed up and I can see Ken getting more and more frustrated. I'm scared that I'll eventually loose him. He's getting ill also! I know he loves me, but how long can a person cope with this uncertainty and stress. We were so hopeful after my cyst was removed last year. We thought we might have found an answer. God, give me the strength to continue. Help me to find answers and the reason why this is happening. I can learn to live with the pain but can't function with the weakness and blackouts."

That afternoon I had an appointment with my doctor. Ken called and said he would drive me there. I was so thankful and hated to always ask for help. The hardest thing about all of this was loosing my independence. As I walked into his office, I quickly sensed that even the receptionist and the nurses were different with me. My doctor just shook his head and said I should return to the first neurologist who had seen me several times. Obviously they were all fed up with seeing my face, not that I could blame them. I sometimes wished that one of my doctors could experience what I had for only a few days to truly understand the situation.

I played my relaxation tape as much as possible and tried to be positive. I didn't watch anything depressing on television. We rented comedies, anything to laugh. I missed being the fun person I had once been. My real self was somewhere inside this monster that had enveloped me. I would shed it! The best way I can express to you how I really felt is to give you direct quotes from my diary.

April 27, 1990 (notes from diary)

I hardly slept last night. I'm having pain throughout my body. My spine hurts from one end to the other. I feel like vomiting. My left side is so sore and, at times, on my right side under my breast. At times it feels like my muscles are turning to stone, I can hardly move. Dear God, please let the neurologist finally help me.

Back again we went to the same neurologist I had seen at the beginning. He again gave me a check-up and said he could not see anything significantly wrong that would give me these symptoms. He assured me he would discuss this with my general practitioner and they would decide if any further testing should be done. He strongly reminded me that I was "focusing" too much on this and I should try to relax. I was more of a mess mentally when I walked out then when I went into his office. I took a Zantac for my stomach and we did the Ben-Gay rub. Ben and I are having quite an affair. Nightly in fact!

I was able to sleep a few hours that night. What wonderful bliss to sleep up to 3 hours at a time. The next morning I tried to start recovering a chair cushion, as I wanted to keep busy. I was so tired and my hands were so sore, I couldn't hold the tools. Okay, if that was too hard then I would try and make cookies. I got all the ingredients out and started to mix the dough but my hands were so sore and were cramping so badly it took forever to get the dough mixed. I managed to surprise Ken and Rachelle with homemade cookies. Terry called again that day and said she had seen a neurologist, who was also interested in my illness. I told her that unless a doctor took my case on as a challenge and kept at it until he found something, nothing would change, I had seen so many doctors by now.

The inevitable has happened. Ken is now on stress medication, a week of stress leave, and his colitis is worse. A condition most likely brought on by all this stress. We seem to be at a standstill. Each time we ask for help, we come up against a brick wall. One thing I have concluded, whatever I have is systemic. I wonder again about lupus. Why on earth can't doctors come together to discuss a case such as this? I was convinced, after going through what I had been through, that others also must be experiencing the same thing. If they worked more as a team it would be most beneficial for some patients. I thought of sending a proposal to the Health Minister, but concluded my letter would most likely stay in a basket and nothing would come out of it.

At this time Rachelle was in horse shows. I tried to attend as much as I could. I would have to make sure the car was close by and I had a chair because I couldn't stand for any length of time. I was so proud of her; she was doing well and coming home with ribbons. As I looked at her, I thought of all the kids and how well they were doing. "Now remember them all when you think you can't take anymore and think of doing something stupid that would hurt them immensely."

As I sit and look out the window at the joggers and families walking, I'm so jealous of them. Inside of me is a person who wants to run and run away from all of this. I'm only 48 years old and I can't even walk four blocks and don't know why. "Here I go again," I think, "self pity!" I know there are others worse off than me and I pray for them and thank God I'm still alive. "But please give us a reason and an explanation," I ask. That's all I was asking for now, I needed to know what I had.

May 1990

The last few weeks I'm getting more swollen and itchy. I wonder if it's my bowels or kidneys. I haven't heard from my general practitioner, the neurologist or the lupus specialist in Calgary. I called the neurologist's office and I'm told he called my general practitioner shortly after seeing me. I called my doctor's office and asked if he could return my call, as I would like to know what the neurologist had said. Knowing how anxious I was to get any feedback, I shouldn't have to call to get the information. But by this time they were not too concerned that I had something of great significance. That evening my general practitioner called and said, "What can I do for you?" I couldn't help but smile and think, "He had a recall problem, as well." I practically lived at his office and had been to emergency twice that month and he still had to ask? Of course, I was told to book an appointment so he could tell me what the neurologist had said. I was hurt and angry that he wouldn't give me the information over the phone. Maybe the information was serious and he wanted to see me in person. I would give him the benefit of the doubt. The way he talked to me I could see he was convinced I must be a hypochondriac and had most likely discussed that with the neurologist. What had the psychiatrist from the Hope Clinic done to me? I guessed it was one conclusion that could be readily accepted if it was in black and white.

I decided to quit taking Aspirin. They didn't seem to be helping any longer and my stomach was very bad. Ken and I went back to the medical office, he to see another doctor and I to see mine. When I walked into his office he said, "What can I do for you?" I teased him and said that line had to be his favorite line. He was not impressed and said, "You know Annette, like I've told you before, after all the doctors that have seen you, if anything was seriously wrong we would have detected it by now." I answered, "I can't help it, something is ravaging my body and it won't go away. I'll find the answer one day and I'll tell you what it is." I told him that I wanted Ken to come in. We went through what was currently happening and how Ken was now ill, as well. We shared with him how we could no longer cope and didn't know what to do. He said the neurologist had not found anything from his exam and felt I was anxious and focusing too much on myself. He ordered more blood test and said, "Let's wait and see what the colonoscopy test results will say and I suggest you both see a psychiatrist."

That week I called the gastroenterologist asking if the test could be done sooner. I was told it was impossible and she gave me a different prescription. None of the pills were working and I had severe attacks to the left side of my bowel. I didn't know what else to do, so I laid down and cried. My diary is filled with prayers of hope. As I read through it now, it is frightening to think of what I might have done were it not for my faith and the love I received.

I was now unable to attend mass very often and missed it terribly. I was torn between trying to go places or not. Usually I couldn't last very long anywhere and had to come home, so I stayed home most of the time.

Ken, in tears, tells me he can't handle the situation any longer. I have known it would only be a matter of time before this happened. I tell him I understand and it might help if he goes away, even to his parents for a while. We couldn't both go crazy, I would have to somehow cope. Rachelle was taking the bus to school so she didn't need a ride. I would arrange for her rides to her music lessons and other outings. She had her Learner's Permit and would soon have her Driver's Licence. My self-esteem is at an all time low. We are holding each other and crying. He decides he can't leave me alone and we would face whatever we had to together. We keep holding each other and pray that God helps us to keep our sanity.

The stress was aggravating both of our conditions. My brother Bernie gave us a relaxation tape that we started listening to in the evening. We decided we had to keep looking after ourselves and take whatever action we could to better the situation. By now my medical library was expanding. I had read about vitamin C and its benefits and started on 2000 to 3000 mg a day. From what I had read, these amounts should not be harmful. At this point anything was worth a try. I could not simply lie there and not do anything and feel sorry for myself. Somehow I would improve the quality of my life and of those around me.

That week I called the Lupus Society. I wasn't sure that's what I had, but I decided it wouldn't hurt to get more information. I was told to contact a doctor at the Humanity Hospital, who was well versed in this disorder. When I called his office I was told I needed a referral and I wasn't surprised, as this was a normal procedure to see a specialist. I phoned my general practitioner's office and I was told I had to come in and see him to get a referral. They knew how hard it was for me to get rides to keep going in to see them because I could no longer drive at this point. Two phone calls could have happened in a matter of a few minutes and my appointment could have been made. I found a ride and sat across his desk while he dictated a letter to this specialist. He indicated I had been to the Hope Clinic, etc., etc. It was clear again what he was implying to this doctor. An appointment was made for me on May 17, the day before the colonoscopy with the gastroentologist.

May 10, 1990 (notes from diary)

Rachelle is 16 years old today. She is a fine young lady and I'm sure will continue to bring us joy, as the others do. I will bake her a cake today for supper and on May 12 we will be celebrating her birthday at Joanne's and Dennis' home, where we will be spoiled with some great cooking.

This morning I got up to go to the bathroom and my heart started pounding in my chest and it felt like blood was gushing to my neck. I went back to bed as quickly as I could. My neck and throat got sore and I had pain in my left ear, then in my left shoulder. Then it spread to the rest of my body and my calves hurt so much. I'm totally congested and so sore! My left side hurts when I cough. God, get me through this day, please. I'm taking Ecotrin for pain and have taken vitamin C for a week now. Maybe I'm taking too much, like my friend thinks. I'm going to continue for a while. Ken is now on stress leave and is working outside as much as possible. I think it's good therapy for him. I only wish I could be there working with him.

In mid May I decided to apply for long-term disability benefits. I had to accept the fact I could no longer work. This, in itself, was devastating to me. I made an appointment with my general practitioner to discuss this and ask him to fill out my form. He said he would fill it and put at the top that I was in my "chronic years." I felt that was pathetic and sexist! I think he could have put that I had a chronic illness that was still being investigated. What would the insurance company think, that I was applying for disability benefits because I was menopausal? I suppose he didn't know what to put, but we could have discussed it before it was filled out.

Ken got more and more aggravated with the situation and would, at times, lash out at me. I knew now he felt I had to be exaggerating. I needed his support and love desperately and I was in turn trying to support him as well. This was like a never-ending circle of stress. Ken was now on his third week of stress leave. His doctor had made a referral to a psychiatrist. I felt things were getting out of hand and didn't know what to do, except blame myself for all of it. At times I would think he was being unfair. After all, other people had to deal with health situations. The only difference was that we didn't know what we were dealing with. Were my expectations of him too high? We concluded that we had to take things one day at a time. I was not too anxious for him to go to the psychiatrist after my fiasco with one. I felt things couldn't get any worse, so they simply had to improve.

I continued to take vitamin C. It had been a few weeks now and at times it seemed like I had a little more strength. I would continue on these but my stomach was so sore and I wondered if I was taking too many. I would no longer ask my doctor about vitamins and minerals, as he did not believe in supplements and told me I would get everything I need from the food I ate.

May 17, 1990

As I was sitting waiting for the colonoscopy, I suddenly started a major phobia of the hospital and felt like running out. Ken helped me get over it and reminded me that we might get answers and help from this test. I had to hang in there. The night before I had to take all the necessary stuff to prepare myself for this test. I was sure I had the cleanest intestines in town! I was given an I.V. and a mild sedative. During the test, I remember a sharp pain and it felt like they were tearing my bowels. The doctor said something and I was put out again. When I awoke, I was told I would be called regarding the results.

Ken went back to work and the days at home alone were long and most of the time frightening. I noticed that the sharp pain in my tummy had left me and was thankful for that. Even walking was very hard at this point. I hesitated to call family and friends any longer for fear that they were fed up with my problems and me. Even so, the need to share was very high and I would write in my diary. Any activities were now very limited. I tried not to talk about it to Rachelle and Ken but, at times, it was out before I could stop it.

That spring we planted some flowers and Ken worked hard to make the yard look nice. Gardening is a love of mine and I missed it terribly. Ken would help me to the flowerbeds and I would sit on the ground with my hand gardening tools and try doing a little work. Everything was turning green, the horses were grazing, and spring had always been a positive time for me. I had to keep that thought; somehow I would find answers. I wanted so much to do what I used to in the spring. House clean, wash off our bikes and take our first spring ride together with the kids, walk, run and laugh.

May 23, 1990

My appointment with the lupus specialist in Edmonton had been changed to this day. Another doctor! I sat across from him and said, "Doctor, I will be candid with you. I'm desperate for help, can you please try and help me?" Being an observant person, I could tell immediately that he was sincere, sympathetic and would truly try to help me. He asked a lot of questions and even gave me time to respond and ask my own questions. Good Lord, he had great communication skills as well.

He examined me—looking a lot at my hands, nails and feet. At that time I had a severe rash on my body. He then asked me if I ever had a 24-hour urine analysis. I answered that I had never had one. He replied, "This is out of my area, but I would like to order blood work and a 24-hour urine test." I was impressed that he didn't say it wasn't lupus and send me on my way.

The next week my mother's friend Teresa came and did reflexology on my feet. She could not believe what I looked like, especially my feet. They were so red, swollen and sore. I could hardly stand her touching them when she tried to work on them. There had to be something else I could try, possibly something natural might help. I had always been skeptical about non-conventional medicine and was not knowledgeable as to where to start. I had to look into it, as conventional medicine was not helping.

June 1990

Ken and I are getting desperate! We have prayed for strength to cope, but now are at a lost. The lupus specialist I had recently seen called me as soon as the blood test results were in and told me it confirmed what he felt, that it was not lupus. He said he would call me as soon as he had the results from the urine analysis. Regardless if he could help me or not, I knew this doctor had chosen the right profession and was honoring the doctor's creed.

The gastroentologist's office called and, as I suspected, made me come in to the office for the results. I waited close to an hour and got to talk to her for about 5 minutes. She informed me I had a twisted bowel and that she was able to straighten it out with the scope to some extent. I told her that the extreme sharp pain had left me and I was thankful for that. I asked her if it might be a result of my last surgery and she couldn't tell me what had caused it to twist. As far as my other symptoms, she said they were most likely not related to her area.

Rachelle was now in Grade 11 and singing in the choir at the Cathedral for the Grade 12 graduation. We decided to attend the mass. After walking from the parking lot and around the block to the church and up a flight of stairs, I felt terrible. I was out of breath, had chest pains, pain in my left arm, left side of the neck and my left thigh. Then the pain started in my right arm and shoulder and I just could not get enough air. I managed to stay for the mass and did not feel well for the rest of the day. Ken was having a heck of a time handling it this time. We didn't know what to do! If we went to emergency, they would put us through the same thing and send us home to deal with the same thing again. The hardest thing about chronic illness is what others have to go through because of it, especially when we don't know what the chronic illness is. I felt powerless to do anything more. At this time I felt I had seen every doctor I could think of that could possibly help me.

When we got home Ken said he was so drained he had to take a nap. My heart felt strange and tight. I decided I had to get in the car and drive into Sherwood Park to a Medi-Centre. It was a most frightening drive because I was so ill. I hadn't even told Ken I was going. I just went. I saw an older doctor and had to tell him some of the history. He felt immediately that whatever I had was affecting my heart or my heart might be causing some of the other problems. He thought it might be angina and had me take an ECG to see if there was indication of a heart attack. He asked if my thyroid had been checked and I told him I presumed so because of all the tests that had been taken, but I wasn't sure. I assured him I would ask my general practitioner when I saw him. The ECG appeared normal and he prescribed Nitroglycerin in case the pain would come back. He told me to tell my doctor about what had happened. I assured him I would and thanked him for his help. As I drove back home, I wondered if Ken was right in wanting to go back to the Hope Clinic again. Where would we get the money? We had talked about selling the home we had recently built. It was a major fight to try and get disability benefits. As with all insurance companies, paying the client is a whole different story than collecting from us.

The next day we went to get groceries. As neither one of us was feeling well enough to go alone, we decided to go in the store together. We were running out of everything and had to get food. During our shopping, we had to leave the cart there and go to the car because Ken started a bad nosebleed. We stayed there for a while until it stopped and went back in to finish. On the way home I started chest pain and decided to take a Nitro. It gave me a headache, but it did take away the pain in my chest, throat and jaw.

My digestion seemed worse, my lungs felt sore and I would hear a "crinkling-like" sound when I would breath deeply. I desperately tried not to focus on my health, but that was virtually impossible. Day after day my goal was to find some answers. Here and there they were finding things, but no one was putting things together or there was serious miscommunication on the part of the doctors.

That week the lupus specialist called to tell me the urine test result did not indicate what he thought it might. He apologized for not being able to help. I was impressed and assured him he had been most helpful by eliminating lupus and showing genuine concern. He also gave me the name of a cardiologist that I should see. I phoned my doctor's office and told them what this specialist had suggested, but I was asked to make an appointment.

I was so ill I couldn't drive any longer and hated being dependent on others. Lorena was kind enough to say she would take me, but couldn't get her car started that day. So I canceled the appointment and asked if the doctor could call me instead. When he called I informed him what the gastroentologist, immunologist and the doctor from the Medi-Centre had said. I also told him that two doctors had suggested I see a cardiologist. He said, "Now Annette, I can't take all of this down in writing so you had better come in and see me and we'll try to book some heart tests." Could nothing happen over the phone with this doctor? The next day I had to call my son Robert and ask if he could take time off to drive me to my appointment. As co-owner of an electronics company, I knew how busy he was and hated to disturb him. I felt I couldn't ask Lois again, as she also worked part-time and had a family to care for. At this point I would not ask Ken, even if it meant taking a taxi. Things were very strained between us and I refused to aggravate the situation any further, if I could help it. Robert called back and said he would be pleased to take me. Thank God for kind and loving children!

My doctor took blood tests, a lung x-ray and an ECG. He said the blood test indicated I had a viral infection and prescribed antibiotic. My understanding was that antibiotic did nothing for a viral infection, but at this point I was not about to argue. He booked an appointment with an older internist who handled cardiology patients at the Sisters of Charity Hospital and also booked me for an echocardiogram. These were booked for July 23 and August 31 respectively. I noted these on my calendar when I got home and thought it was a long time to wait for these appointments. I know that this poor doctor knew there was something wrong but just couldn't get to the bottom of it.

Ken was not happy with the news and said, "Why don't they just take a CAT scan of your body and be done with it, can't they understand we need help?" It tore me apart to see him so hurt and frustrated. My hope for help and a cure was dwindling.

The next day mom and her friend Teresa came over. She gave me a hand, arm and foot massage and was surprised at the lumps I had in my arms. She left me a book about God's spirit guiding our way and our health. I read it and it once again renewed my faith and I was willing to go on a day at a time and see what would happen.

June 8, 1990

When I got up and looked outside, the sun was shinning and I decided to go outside and try to do a little work in the garden. I just had to try. I sat by the edge and did a little weeding for about half an hour. I was out of breath but determined to continue. I went in and sat for a while in the kitchen before continuing to the bedroom. I had a shower and then decided to make some squares and surprise Ken. I was mixing the batter with great difficulty when my upper back got very sore, as did my arms and legs. My thumbs and first fingers cramped up and I could not straighten them. The pain in my upper back got very bad and I started to shake. I got pain in my neck and left side of my face, then numbness in my left hand and side of the face. I was so frightened; I didn't know what to do. I put my hands under hot water and tried to massage them. Finally, I was able to move them again.

I got mad at God and started screaming at him and asking him what he thought he was doing to me. Ken called about this time and asked me how my day was going. I shared it with him and I could tell he was feeling the pain and anguish also. I was so weak; I had to lie down and I cried. I couldn't drive myself anywhere, but I was not about to ask anyone to drive me. If I were to die right there, then I wouldn't have to deal with it any more.

In the evening I wrote in my diary, hardly able to hold the pen for the pain in my back and arms. Trying to do a little work that day resulted in the pain being even worse. My diary that night reads, "It has been a very bad day. I have suffered for so long that I fear what the outcome may be, even if someone does diagnose my illness." I watched the sun set like I have for so many nights. The horses were grazing and it looked so peaceful. I so desperately want to grab that peace and hold on to it and carry it to my body as a healer. I questioned God every night and asked him to help me carry this burden I had been given. What was his reason for this?

June 9, 1990

Last night was a very bad night. I stayed up most of the night in the living room. Ken went to bring Rachelle to her music lesson about 9:00 a.m. I got up and went to get meat out of the deepfreeze. I felt so weak that I had to go back to bed. As I passed the living room, I knew I was blacking out and headed for the phone by our bed. I dialed 911 and started to tell her what was wrong and managed to tell her where we lived. She kept talking to me, but she sounded far away. I don't remember anything after that, except someone was talking close to my face and an I.V. was being inserted. I also remember them talking to me in the ambulance off and on.

I was brought to the Sisters of Charity Hospital. All the usual things were done—like blood pressure, blood tests and my history were taken again. A cardiologist intern came in to see me with another doctor. The last doctor that came in looked at my hands and feet and asked me if I smoked. I told him I had never smoked and wondered why he had asked. "You look like you have Raynaud's phenomenon and inflammation of the chest." I was booked into the hospital about 3 p.m.

The night was long! What was I doing in a hospital again? Perhaps I shouldn't have called for help. I felt so frightened and lonely. The loud zinging sensation and noise came again just before I fell asleep.

The next morning my general practitioner came in, looked at me and said, "You two had better get your stories straight." I could not believe what he had said and did not know what in the world he was talking about. He thought I had told the cardiologist I thought I had a heart problem. I had said no such thing, except for saying that two doctors had suggested I see a cardiologist. Where in the world did he get an idea like that? Ken was mad that he had insinuated such a thing. In the event I had said something I shouldn't have, I apologized to end this ridiculous conversation. We think he was just annoyed that I had not tried to contact him before going to emergency. He had some good points about him, but he was young and had a lot to learn before becoming the humanitarian that doctors pledge to be. It still never ceases to amaze me how doctors don't listen to their patients and could eliminate problems by doing so.

Ken, Rachelle and Joanne came to visit in the afternoon. If only they knew how nice it was to see them. Rachelle brought me her Chip and Dale playing cards and we all laughed about this. "Mom, since your such a sexy French lady, you might enjoy these when you play solitaire," said Rachelle. "I wonder what has happened to that sensual French lady?" I said. What was ravaging my body to change me so much? A neurologist intern then came in to talk to and check me.

That evening Lois, my neighbor, and Robert, Lorena and Daniel came to see me. They were concerned and I couldn't provide any more answers than before. I looked at Daniel and hoped I would see him grow up. We had a nice time together and talked a lot about how fast the baby was growing and of all the new things he was learning. As they left, I wanted to be with them and walk out and go home. It was so hard to be in this room alone again. I was given an anti-inflammatory drug called Orudis E and two extra-strength Tylenol that night.

The same thing happened as I fell asleep last night. Also, during the night I woke up with a strange sensation with pain in the back of my head. I felt like I was far away and couldn't wake up. I got up to go to the bathroom and when I came back to bed my heart was racing.

The next morning I had some breakfast and the I.V. was taken out. I had a shower and the warm water felt good. I closed my eyes and pretended we were on holidays and I was getting ready to go sightseeing. The tears fell, mixing with the water. Just deal with today and see what tomorrow brings I told myself.

My doctor was in and said, "Well, the neurologist did not find anything wrong during his examination but he wants to do some tests." He told me he would get back to me later and after this test was done, the others could be done as an outpatient. I was hooked up to a 24-hour Holter tape to monitor my heart. I felt very ill that day and evening.

June 12, 1990

The days pass slowly and I look outside at "normal" people walking around and I pray one day I can again be like them. I am taken down for an evoke response test and an echocardiogram. The evoke response test is normal and I have to wait for the other results. I was certainly finding out what wasn't wrong with me anyhow! It would probably be an elimination game all the way.

Mom and her friend Teresa came in to see me. She massaged my feet and they felt much warmer. My feet and legs were like ice, which was different for me because they were usually red and swollen. Around lunchtime my feet and hands went numb and tingly. I felt very ill and nauseated. It is most likely needless to elaborate how depressed I was at this time. A student nurse in her 30's came in and sat down and started talking about other ways of healing. I was surprised to hear this from someone who wanted to be a nurse in conventional medicine. I found out that she wanted her nursing to compliment her knowledge of natural healing. She was informed on acupressure and asked if I would mind if she worked on my back. Was I dreaming this? Was she an angel who had come because of my prayers?

She rubbed my back with Tiger Balm that she had with her. It surprised her to see the condition of my back and neck muscles. With the pain I was experiencing, she was unable to work very much, but even the warmth of the balm felt so good. We both knew this was "unorthodox" and would keep it to ourselves. It was most gratifying to get any kind of relief from pain and discomfort.

The neurologist intern was in with a senior neurologist. They looked at my legs and were bewildered with all the involuntary movements that they called vasiculation. I was told I would have to go through a few more tests. Neurological tests were usually painful. If it was neurological, then why hadn't it been found before? I have had so many tests; surely something would have been noticed. God I was scared and fed up! If my legs could have carried me, I would have walked out that night. To what, or where, I don't know, I just wanted to get out so badly.

At my lowest point that day, the student nurse from the previous day came to see me after her shift. We talked about positive thinking and positive attitudes, and about thinking that I would be healed. After she left, the next hours were spent in prayer for strength. After all, there had to be a reason for this in my life and who was I to question God's plan for me.

June 13, 1990

Today I would get my neurological muscle test. I had a similar test at the Hope Clinic, so I knew what I was in for. More pain, more needles. There was a knock at the door and a minister walked in. He was a great listener and we talked about expectations of others and ourselves. I was able to cry and share my frustrations. God had sent him at a most appropriate time! I don't recall his name, but I will never forget his kindness. He told me he had once been a truck driver, which goes to show there are some pretty nice truck drivers out there. My neighbor Lois said she would bring me down to my test and wait with me. It was my good fortune she was with me as we waited an hour. I couldn't believe that these people had come to me when I so desperately needed them.

The test was painful as I suspected. In the afternoon I had company, which helped pass the time. In the evening Ken, Rachelle, Robert, Lorena and Daniel came for a while. That was great and helped the evening go by. The student nurse stopped in while Ken was there and left some Tiger Balm with him. Before leaving, he rubbed my back and it was soothing and special, I missed his gentle touch. I closed my eyes and fell asleep smelling balm mixed with the smell of all the flowers.

July 14, 1990

I woke up very congested and was having trouble breathing. My hands and face felt numb. What a weird sensation. Why was I so out of breath? I explained this to the nurse and I was given oxygen that helped immediately. Mom came up and stayed with me for the rest of the afternoon and into the evening. I was so grateful to her for being there. My doctor came in later in the evening and said, "Most of your tests are okay. The neurologist seems to think you might be hyperventilating." I said that I doubted my congestion and lack of oxygen was due to hyper-ventilation. He said, "They saw a fluid pocket by the heart. The doctor feels it will probably dissipate on it's own, but that it shouldn't be causing all of your symptoms." I answered, "If it's hyperventilation, I suggest we get a psy-chiatrist in here to clarify this once and for all!" He felt I was getting defensive. I added that at this point I was basically non-functional and would not leave the hospital before someone could determine what in the hell I had and how it could be treated. I could see he was stunned by my reaction, as it was out of character of me to be so assertive. I knew he was confused as well, but he had to realize the incredible frustration we were going through.

Joanne was in for a visit and was as supportive as ever, always trying to cheer me up. Rachelle came in with anoth-er Danielle Steel book and to tell me she had passed her Driver's test. She was growing up too quickly! My girlfriend Linda and I talked on the phone for awhile. Thank God for special people! My sister Terry later called from Montreal. I'm sure her phone bill is outrageous. We talk and wonder about the genetic thing again. One doctor has recently told her that she most likely has a connective tissue disease. I went to sleep with the oxygen on and this really bewildered me. I'd been congested before, but never felt like this.

The next day my doctor came in and said the liver blood tests were normal and the blood gases showed high alkaline, which could be blocking the calcium. He added that the doctor handling cardiology felt there was nothing wrong with my cardiovascular system. Also, that they were unable to confirm a diagnosis as to a connective tissue disorder. We talked about a biopsy but he felt the lumps were not large enough. I couldn't figure out that answer because my whole left side was lumpy. A psychiatrist will see me soon. Hopefully, he might shed some light on a few things. I was uneasy, to say the least, about this visit after my first experience with one. Whatever the outcome, I would have a report sent to my doctor.

Ken and I talked on the phone and we couldn't even talk about the current situation anymore. I knew if somehow I didn't get some answers, I would have a broken marriage. How would I ever deal with something like that, as well as this illness?

I had quite a few visitors and was extremely tired. I was still on oxygen, which was a complete mystery. I had been in this room for 6 days. I decided I would ask someone to wheel me out of this room tomorrow. My ankles were really swollen so I asked Ken to bring me some grapefruit, as I had read that they were a natural diuretic.

June 16, 1990

I spent a terribly long night. My spine was very sore and so were my joints. I was out of breath and shaky. I decided to get up and walk around the room to keep up some kind of strength. I was ever thankful for the company of my books; they kept me sane for years. I did some positive imagery and talked to my sisters Terry and Michelle on the phone. Ken came in and I put my best attitude on. I decided to walk to the kitchen without the oxygen and when I came back to the room, my whole body felt strange. I felt weak and shaky, my chest felt tight and my arms and back hurt. I was so very discouraged. The pulsating in my left ear was very loud. Ken looked so down, we started to cry. We were holding hands and he noticed they were turning blue. He called the nurse who gave me oxygen and Ativan. I presumed the Ativan was to calm me down. Ken stayed for a while and we just sat there together, not saying anything. What could we say!

June 17, 1990 (Father's Day)

The family came to visit and everyone is concerned and wondering how long it will take before we get some answers. How unfair this is for everyone! I was fortunate to receive Holy Communion almost daily. I was thankful for the faith my parents had provided for me. Ken and Rachelle took me for a ride in a wheelchair. It was not long after I was out of the room that I noticed I could breathe better. We concluded that it must be something in my room that was causing this. When I returned to my room I had to put the oxygen back on. I would have to mention this to the doctor. I fell asleep while looking at the picture of my children, holding a letter Rachelle had just given me, and looking out the window at the setting sun. How had I rated a room that let me see the sun set? I don't know, but I was thankful for it.

June 18, 1990

Another day, and I begin to understand what courage it must take to be confined to this life forever. The psychiatrist came and we discussed everything that had been happening to me. He was a totally different human being. After a long talk, he indicated he did not feel it was psychological. I wasn't surprised at his conclusion, but was glad a report would note that fact. He was interested in the car accident and said the severe impact could have damaged blood vessels, which could not be seen on a CAT scan and suggested another type of scan. He added it was no wonder we were stressed after 6 years of living this hell. He said he would arrange for the scan.

Friends, family and co-workers came bearing gifts and flowers. Their visits and kindness was much appreciated. My doctor came in and we discussed what the psychologist had said. He added it might be a good idea to prescribe something for the anxiety. I feel so sorry for him; he seems at such a loss. I begin to question my expectation regarding the medical profession. Joanne stopped by and brought me books on yeast syndrome and acupressure. I devour these in hopes of finding answers.

After company left that day, I watered the flowers and walked a bit around the room. After about 10 minutes, my chest felt tight and breathing was difficult. My throat felt funny and my left arm hurt and after a while, my right arm. I could breath much better after I laid down and took oxygen. "What the heck is going on?" I thought. I decided it was okay to get mad and cry. I wanted to throw things around. I cried until I could cry no more. "So much for my positive thinking," I thought. That night my prayer was, "God, please, have your forgotten me? Don't abandon me, please, please. Let me know why I have to go through this. Keep my family and friends healthy so that they may never have to go through pain and discomfort like this."

The next day was spent much the same. A couple of girls from work came to see me and we had some good laughs, something I didn't do too much lately. While laughing, I suddenly felt a sudden sharp pain in my left chest cavity. My ears felt very warm and were "popping." It was quite amazing because after that, I had a quiet kind of feeling in my body. I wondered what had happened? Whatever it was, I told the girls they would have to come back and make me laugh again. After they left I wondered if it was the anti-inflammatory pills or the calcium that suddenly made my body feel this way. Was it something to do with the fluid on the heart? It couldn't be the anti-anxiety pills, as I had not been given any yet. That night, although I had to use the oxygen, I had less pain and hardly any pulsating. My body felt so strange, so quite. I was sure I had died and gone to heaven. I hadn't felt like this in a long, long time. I thanked God for giving me this time with less pain and asked if I could have more relief.

The following day I had company and the psychiatrist came by and asked that I make an appointment with him in a few weeks. He felt he might be able to help me deal with this ongoing illness. I seemed to have less pain today. Were the anti-inflammatory pills doing something?

June 21, 1990

It is the first day of summer and it looks so beautiful outside! I'm very congested and have to keep the oxygen on all the time today. My friend Hélène was in to visit. We talked about how she had struggled with fatigue for years and couldn't find answers. How unfair it was to her and her family. After she leaves, I feel so grateful for the time she has taken to visit with me. My doctor came in and said I would see a lung specialist. The need for oxygen really bewildered him also. That evening Ken and all the kids were in to see me and I wasn't able to put on a very good act. I broke down and cried and shared with them how I wanted to go home.

On June 22 I had a head scan, which would indicate the amount of blood flow to the brain. As I was going through this, I wondered what happened to all the radioactive material that was put into my body with all these tests. The lung specialist's assistant came in and listened to my lungs and talked to me. The specialist came in briefly. I wanted to ask some questions but was abruptly interrupted. A lung test was scheduled. I can't imagine why I'm so darn out of breath in this hospital. This has never happened to me before!

Ken came in and told me he had seen a psychiatrist yesterday and it was quite a joke. He told him he didn't do stress management, so Ken told him "I guess you can't help me because stress is my problem." He wouldn't even take the time to let Ken vent his frustrations or give him direction. What in the world did this psychiatrist treat, if stress wasn't included? What did he collect Alberta Health Care money for? Ken was not impressed, to say the least, and it would be difficult to get him to see anyone else.

We went downstairs for a while and had a nice visit. At times we felt so close. I guess we had been through so much that if we could hang in there together, we would be even closer. We felt positive that night that somehow we would get answers. Thank God for the positive times! He wheeled me out on the terrace and it felt like a great gift. I could breathe much better out there; in fact, I could breath much better out of my room period. This was the third time I had felt I could breathe better out of that room. Something in there had to be causing it!

We went back to my room and looked around to see what could possibly be causing this. As I walked towards the window, I started gasping for air. Right next to me were flowers. "The flowers," I said, "could it be the flowers?" Numerous times I have had flowers around me, why would they bother me so much this time? I sniffed them up close and when I got to a beautiful large bouquet with lilies, my throat felt funny and I felt like I was choking. "My God, all this time it must have been the flowers!" We put them all in the bathroom to see what would happen.

That night I needed less oxygen and told my doctor about it when he came in the next morning. He seemed very unimpressed and said, "The lung specialist doesn't think you have asthma." He asked me if I would like to go home. I told him I missed home terribly, but I was a little frightened to do so because I was so very weak. "Well then, we'll see tomorrow," he said. When he walked out I vowed that one day I would find out what this monster was and when I did, I would find ways to improve this condition and shout it to the world! No way would I give up. No way!

June 24, 1990

Had I really been here 14 days? At times I pretended it was all a bad dream and I would soon wake up from it. I told Ken to go to the lake with the kids. Poor guy, he needed something else to do on a Sunday other than to be here again. I was told I would have my lung function test on Monday. I have sent the flowers home and can breath much better now. I prayed and read for most of the day. John and Linda came to visit which was most appreciated. It was a long, long day.

June 25, 1990

I slept fairly well last night, but towards morning I had loud, swishing, pulsating noises and a "weird" sensation in my upper back and it spread to my limbs. What was new? These things had been happening to me for over 5 years now. My doctor told me I could go home today and to come back tomorrow for a thallium stress test (for coronary artery blockage). He gave me a prescription for Ventolin, Orudis and calcium. I was to see him the next week for the results. I then went down for the pulmonary function test and the lab technologist said it looked okay. I presumed I had been right, that it was an allergic reaction to the flowers. Ken said he would pick me up at 4:30. I packed and knew I would only survive with a positive attitude. Things would surely improve; after all, I could walk around a bit now.

When we walked into our house, again it seemed so large and bright after all that time in a hospital room. When I walked into the bedroom, memories flooded back when I had last been here. "That's all right," I said, "it's in the past and it won't happen again."

The following morning we were at the hospital at 7:15 a.m. for the stress test. The nurse who put in the I.V. hurt me so much that I cried. I don't know what she did because I had had many before and none had ever hurt as much. She looked at me and said, "Now, does it really hurt that much?" The test was hard for me because they made me walk on a treadmill. I could barely finish what they asked me to do.

After the test Ken and I stopped for a burger. It was like going out on a great outing. It had been so long since we had been out anywhere. He stopped to look at a garden tractor that was perfect for us, but we couldn't consider it at this time. Disability benefits are still an ongoing battle. Bernie, May and family came to visit and brought Mom who would stay for a few days. At 77 she was doing well for her age, but I worried she would over do things and asked her to be there for company but not to do any work.

July 1, 1990

I have been home for 6 days now. Some of them had not been too bad and others were not good. I look at Ken working outside and want to be out there working with him. I sometimes sit outside and feel so useless. Financially this illness has been disastrous. At times I say it's my fault and Ken gets annoyed at me for saying this. I tried to do as much as possible around the house. The accomplishments, no matter how small, were psychologically beneficial.

A nun from the orphanage where we helped at Christmas, told us about a holistic chiropractor that had helped her a lot. I decided I would call her and see what the charges would be. I also made another appointment with the psychiatrist who had recently seen me at the hospital. His reassurance that "it was not all in my head" helped me cope. It helped to be able to talk to someone like him because things at home were very stressed. Lately, Ken had a very short fuse. He would get mad and say things like, "All we talk about is this stupid illness and doctors around here now." Poor him, we talked about other things but under the circumstances he was right, the illness was the major topic of conversation. If I got defensive, things were only worse so I tried to walk away from the situation when it got too stressed and at times he would be annoyed at this. What a terrible time we were going through. I felt loved one day and not the next. I was so frightened and lonely at times. One of the things that frightened me the most was the state of our relationship. I was sure he felt cheated by what had happened to the person he had married. I think at this time he was worse off emotionally than I was. All kinds of things would run through my head and I started to wonder if at times he would prefer that I died. Then I scolded myself and said, "Stop it, we love each other and will get through this somehow. I had shared a home and family with him for 10 years." I concluded that if I tried hard to cope with this, then others who loved me would have to try also, no matter how hard it was. I was ill and that was that! Had I not done everything possible trying to get help and answers?

When I returned to my general practitioner's office, he informed me that the latest scan indicated some narrowing but no damage to the blood vessels in the neck. We discussed the possibility that this long-term illness could be viral and he seemed to agree that it could be. He told me to "take it easy" and to come back in 3 weeks to see him. I left feeling positive. I had been working so hard on being positive lately. I reminded myself that even if I had this illness that I was an "okay" person. I thanked God for his help and the courage that I needed to keep going.

July 12, 1990 (notes from diary)

I have been trying to walk a bit more lately. I'm scared I'll lose all my strength. Things are better between Ken and I. My doctor had called saying the assisting cardiologist had found something in the upper chamber of my heart and he would get the senior doctor to look at it and get back to us. "My God, are we finally going to get answers?" I said. "What is wrong with my heart and why wasn't it seen in the angiogram at the Humanity Hospital?" At 4:30 p.m. he called again to tell me that the older doctor had not had a chance to look at it, but he thought there was a chance it was a false positive because it sometimes happened in women. "What did they mean?" One minute my doctor is very worried that there is something wrong and, the next, this old doctor says that there isn't without even looking at the test results! He added that this older doctor did not think I needed medication at this time but should be watched closely. This does not make sense, as I know they are both going on holidays this week.

On Saturday I went with Ken to Rachelle's horse show. She had attended a horse clinic that week and now it was time for the concluding events. She was great and won 2 first-places and a second-place. The distraction was so nice even if I was totally exhausted when I got home. I had a very bad night with severe joint and muscle pain, tightness in the chest and indigestion. On Sunday I didn't want to stay alone so I went with Ken to pick up a horse for a friend. I felt so ill that I had to stay in the truck. I had chest pain, nausea and pain in my arms. Ken dropped me off at home and went to bring our friend's horse home. I was so very ill that Rachelle took me to the hospital. All the way I kept thinking that this couldn't be happening. Was a virus killing me? How could Rachelle stand bringing me back to a hospital again and wait for hours in an emergency ward?

I was finally seen by another cardiology resident. After the usual questions, blood gases, x-rays and blood work were done he returned and prescribed Isordil (a longer lasting Nitro pill). He told me to go back to my general practitioner for a follow-up. "Why was everyone giving me Nitro when apparently I had nothing wrong with my heart?" Was a virus damaging my heart? I kept asking myself these questions. That evening Rachelle had a friend over for supper. Ken barbecued some ribs and the girls made salad and vegetables. I wasn't hungry and attempted to keep up with the conversation and ate a few bites.

On Monday I was still very ill and took half a Nitro three times as directed. I phoned to see if I could talk to the cardiologist resident that I had recently seen in emergency, but was told he was unavailable. They let me speak to another resident who said he couldn't help me and abruptly put me back to the operator. I phoned the young cardiologist who had initially felt the test results indicated I had a heart problem. I was told he was on holidays. It seems like everyone that I needed to speak with was on holidays at the same time.

As I lay in bed that morning, I wondered how in this day and age something like this could ever happen to a person. How in the world could it be that no one could come to some consensus and conclusions about this illness? I was so sore and weak that morning I could hardly make it to the bathroom. I prayed again for strength and help. Lois, my neighbor and friend, told me to call her anytime, but I hesitate because she is working most of this week. My stomach is so much worse and I wonder if it's the medication. Rachelle reminded me that it sometimes had to get worse before it got better and that I would see my rainbow. I can't tell her enough how a few words like those keep me going. I called my insurance company and was told there was a possibility that I might get financial help. They would get back to me.

The cardiologist resident, who had seen me in emergency, read the stress test results. He said the report indicated something was malfunctioning because the amount of oxygen needed by my body wasn't being released. He said he would talk to my general practitioner about this, if I wanted him to. I assured him I would be thankful if he would. "Did this account for all the muscle soreness and cramping?" I thought. Why hadn't someone followed this up before? Was it because I was female that the older doctor said it was probably a false positive? Was this some kind of sexist thing again? God, I'm so confused!

July 18, 1990

I got up slowly and after washing I started to walk to the kitchen. My legs started hurting, I felt weak and my heart was pounding. I had chest pain and my jaws, face and neck hurt. I went back to bed because I knew I would land up on the floor again. I closed my eyes wishing I would go to sleep and never wake up again. Rachelle and her girlfriend were home that morning. I called her and told her to call Lois. Lois came over and called an ambulance. She then held me while I cried in desperation. Rachelle was beyond herself and was in tears. Lois tried to reassure her that things would be okay. What terrible stress I was imposing on others! I was taken to the Humanity Hospital because the Sisters of Charity emergency was full. All this time I felt like I was in a fog, there, but not there.

When Ken came to the hospital he was in a state of panic. No wonder he had developed colitis after all we had been through and still had to cope with. I was given oxygen and it seemed to help some of the symptoms. Again they took blood and did an arterial blood test that hurt incredibly and left huge bruises. Then I had a chest x-ray and an ECG. The blood gasses showed I had enough oxygen in my body, but when they took me off oxygen the symptoms started again. I was given a lung scan and it showed I was taking in enough air and it appeared to be "mixing" okay. I must ask my readers to bear with me regarding my lack of medical terminology.

The resident cardiologist showed genuine concern and gave us as much time as we needed to ask questions. He answered our questions, as thoroughly as possible and in a way we could understand. He was in agreement that something was definitely wrong and said he would talk to the doctor at the Sisters of Charity Hospital. After he had contacted him, he told us the thallium stress test was okay as far as the treadmill walk indicated. There was a question, however, in regards to the other part of the test that looks at the heart muscles. He said reading the results were quite subjective and unless he saw the x-rays he couldn't elaborate on the results. All he could do was tell me to take Nitro only when I felt I needed them. He said these would also help the esophagus spasms.

We left the hospital frightened once again knowing that we were no further ahead with this rotten illness. The hospital resident had told us to follow up with our general practitioner the next day, if possible.

July 19, 1990

The follow-up appointment was made with my general practitioner's partner who was replacing mine during his holidays. I explained what had happened and that I just simply couldn't keep going on like this any longer. The left side of my face and head hurt so they felt I should have a sinus x-ray. I asked about toxin tests as well. I also asked if they could set up an appointment with the first young cardiologist who had seen me at the Sisters of Charity Hospital. Also, I wanted an appointment with both the Sisters of

99

Charity's neurologist, who had seen me while I was there, and the gastroentologist. I continued to say that I would start from scratch, if I had to. After all this, he told me I would have to wait until my doctor returned from holidays, as he knew my case much better.

At the receptionist desk, I asked her to make an appointment with the neurologist. She didn't even argue when she looked at me, she picked up the phone and dialed. After the sinus x-ray I called the gastroenterologist to make an appointment. My stomach was so bad I no longer knew what to take. I couldn't digest anything and kept burping. I also made an appointment with the holistic chiropractor. I had to take charge of my situation even if it meant being more assertive.

Ken called his doctor again about a medical leave. He is having trouble sleeping now and his colitis is bad. I can't stand seeing him like this. It's tearing me apart! He desperately has to get away from this situation to get his health back and keep his sanity. He took a week off, until the 30th. His superiors are not as supportive as mine are. How can people be so inconsiderate?

On Friday I stayed in bed until I had to leave for my consultation appointment with the holistic chiropractor. I had never been to a chiropractor in my life and, least of all, not a holistic one. I was skeptical and scared. At this time Medical Care did not include anything but conventional medicine. She seemed caring and felt I might have an absorption problem. She took some x-rays and I left after paying $80 and having made an appointment for Monday.

Saturday was a terrible day! I had pressure on my throat, neck and chest and had trouble breathing. I could not digest anything and felt like fainting. The left side of my face felt sore and I had trouble walking. My whole body ached. It was another long night.

On Sunday we decided to go to the lake with the children. If I was going to feel like this, I might as well be with them and get some distraction. I also didn't want to stay home alone. I sat most of the day and watched the kids waterskiing and Daniel playing in the sand and running around so full of life. As I watched them, I was thankful again for the gifts that God had given me. The children and Ken barbecued and I ate a small piece of steak and a few vegetables, which I suffered for later. I was up most of the night trying everything and anything that might stop the stomach pain and help me burp.

The day had arrived to have my first treatment with the holistic chiropractor. She did tests that I didn't understand. I felt like I was in the hands of a medicine woman. She then showed me my x-rays and pointed to how my back was more curved than it should be. As she worked on my back and neck, I thought, "You wanted to end it all, this will probably do it. With all this cracking she'll surely kill me." The first visit to a chiropractor is quite an experience. As the visit progressed, and so far I had survived, she made me hold a bottle of calcium pills and a bottle of phosphoric acid in each hand. As I held these, she would push down on my arms (energy testing, which I had no clue about at the time). "Good Lord, what had I gotten myself into?" I said to myself. As I left she said, "Now, remember to keep a positive attitude." I wondered how long she would stay positive in my shoes. This appointment cost $70 with the phosphoric acid that I was to take for my stomach. My hopes were up as I left and thought about thinking positive once again. I wasn't sure how long we could afford these visits at these prices.

July 24, 1990

That night I slept a little better. By now I was so sleep deprived, I was like a walking zombie. I still had a lot of trouble with my stomach. I imagined it would take a few days before the phosphoric acid would work. As the day progressed, I seemed to get considerably worse. I called the gastroenterologist to see if I could get into her earlier than August 9. The receptionist said, "I don't think we can see you, we're very busy. If you get worse, go to emergency." Why could they not keep an appointment open for emergency situations? Did they not know how long 2 weeks was when a day seemed like an eternity?

July 25, 1990

I had another terrible night with the same symptoms. My stomach seems as if it's now on fire. Ken went to sleep in the guestroom. I can't blame him. I don't know how he can stand all this. I'm so torn as to what to do next. Should I cancel my appointment with the holistic chiropractor, as the phosphoric acid she gave me seems to be making my stomach much worse? I tried to get a hold of the psychiatrist because I think I'm now on the brink of insanity. I left a message for him. In desperation, I went to the Medi-Centre to ask a doctor to give me a B12 shot in the event it might help. He said he wouldn't give it to me because it might interfere with absorption tests. Back home, I called the gastroenterologist again and begged, in tears, to see the doctor. The receptionist said she would talk to her when she returned to the office. "Please God, let her see me today and help me," I prayed. The receptionist called back saying I had been booked for a gastroscopy on August 7, which seemed like a lifetime away.

I decided to cut the phosphoric acid to 5 drops a meal to see if the burning would lessen. At times, I would look into the mirror and say, "I'm well, I'm not sick." The image that looked back at me told me differently. We went into the empty church and wept. "Why was this happening?" I asked. I needed answers and strength to stop me from going insane. Both Ken and I needed his love now more than ever. I had no doubt in the power and love of God. I felt again that he had his reasons to give me this cross to bear. I was beginning to believe that his reason was that I would somehow help others.

July 27, 1990

I went back to the chiropractor. After all I couldn't be a quitter; didn't she say I most likely had an absorption problem and had given me the phosphoric acid. I was not in good spirits when she first saw me for obvious reasons. Life was not fun and I told her so. "If your stomach is burning so much then you probably have ulcers," she said. "We have to get to the bottom of this." I told her it was like a big ball. I couldn't do anything because of it. I wasn't getting answers and, therefore, was stressed. I was certain the stress was aggravating my symptoms. It was a vicious circle. I had made another appointment with the psychiatrist to see if he could help me cope.

We looked at some x-rays from the Sisters of Charity Hospital. She said that I had compressed disks in the upper spine and a lot of arthritis in the lower back. I had been told recently that I had osteoarthritis in the neck area. She worked on my neck and suggested I continue taking three calcium pills (Re-Cal B that contained different kinds of calcium). The bill was $14, as Health Care would cover the remainder. I came out feeling a little better emotionally, which I felt was very important. I needed anything I could grasp that would trigger positive feelings. Ken and I went for lunch. Our outings, no matter how small, were now far and few between. This was special.

After lunch we left for the psychiatrist appointment. I found him to be as nice as always. I was able to talk to him about the frustrations surrounding my illness. "I sense that you have lost confidence in doctors at this time," he said. I shared that I had experienced a lack of communication between doctor and patient, and between doctors themselves. Often they didn't consider the patient's point of view and lacked awareness regarding the consequences to tests, hospitalization, drugs, etc. I added that I had great respect and admiration for the things that doctors did and also reminded him I was not generalizing when saying such things. He agreed to most of this and proceeded to explain how he worked with patients. There were things like psychotherapy, psychotherapy with drugs, drugs, and even shock treatments, if necessary. As he went on, I could feel myself sinking deeper into the chair and kept one eye on the door. I then remembered the woman who had walked out as I waited for my appointment. She looked like a zombie. Would I become one also? My sense of humor took over again and I visualized myself hooked up to all kinds of electrodes; this in addition to everything else I was coping with. I would refuse drugs because I knew at this point that I could become addicted easily. Being in a cloud instead of having to deal with this could become an easy choice. He suggested I return and we would talk again.

That afternoon Ken's parents came to visit. She shared how iron pills and B12 had helped her. It took a lot to try and visit, I was so ill. My stomach and throat were very bad and I was generally feeling miserable. My legs were so bad; it looked like I had worms crawling inside my calves.

The next morning I asked Rachelle to buy me some iron pills. I was grasping at anything that might give me some relief. Something had to be missing in my body to make it feel like this. When she returned I took one with lunch and then another at night. That was a bad move. My stomach was so bad I wanted to crawl in a hole and die.

On Sunday I went with Rachelle and Ken to a horse show. As hard as it was to drag myself around, I was determined to keep going. Better to be with people than alone at home. I sat in the shade most of the day and looked at others walking from one end of the ring to the other and thought again of how we so often take things for granted. I remember having to go to the bathroom and looking at the outhouse that seemed so far away. I held on for a couple more hours, but decided I had to try it and hoped I would make it without fainting, falling or making a spectacle of myself. I made it having to stop twice to rest on the way. Once inside I cried because now I had to try and make it back to my chair. At lunch I took a calcium tablet and rested in the truck. As usual, Rachelle rode very well and it was such a thrill to watch her and her horse "Personality Plus."

On Monday I returned to the chiropractor. I had slept quite well and was thankful for the few hours of relief. It was not that I couldn't get to sleep; I slept as soon as my head hit the pillow, as I was always so tired. The problem was the pain and discomfort would wake me up and keep me awake most nights. As she worked on me, she again reminded me that I was to try and help myself first and stop worrying about how difficult this was on others. She said in order to help myself; I had to be a little selfish for now. This was my third visit and I still had to get used to all the cracking noise that went on when she worked on me. I was concerned about what all this might do to my spine with the arthritis in it. I was surprised that indeed I did experience some pain relief for a time after she would work on me. Afterwards we stopped at a clothing store but I was exhausted after only a little while. Nevertheless, to me, I had achieved a milestone. We stopped at the park and sat and talked, making it an enjoyable day.

The day of my appointment with the elderly internal medicine specialist who was in charge of cardiology at the Sisters of Charity Hospital was finally here. The receptionist looked at me and said, "Why weren't you here at 9:30 for your appointment?" I answered, "I'm sorry, but it was for 2:30 p.m., there must be some mistake." She replied, "The mistake is yours, not ours. I'm sorry he can't see you." I couldn't believe it. I had put down the date and time when I had last spoke with her and had repeated it to her before hanging up. How could this be happening? I was reminded again that he could not see me and that I would have to rebook for August 30, one month away. I asked her if it would be possible to talk to him on the phone in the near future. I was told he would also be too busy to talk to me on the phone and, regardless, she added, it would be much better to see him. On the way home Rachelle had to deal with a crying mother. She said, "Mom, remember how you always tell us to make the best out of a situation, now you'll have to try and make the best out of this and wait until the 30th, there's nothing you can do, you tried." She was right, and I was proud of her words of wisdom at such a young age. I would just have to wait the month out. I decided I couldn't dwell on it.

When we were making supper I felt just a little bit stronger. It wasn't much but it was there. I wondered if it could be the calcium and vitamin C that I had just started taking. Even a small improvement was like a miracle these days.

My general practitioner was seeing patients that evening. We left for my appointment with the information from the chiropractor. We talked about the stress test results and my visits to the psychiatrist and Medi-Centre. I told him I had taken four iron pills so far. We discussed anemia, B12 and folic acid deficiencies. He didn't comment too much and said he would do blood work for anemia. That evening the pain and discomfort didn't seem quite as severe. This time I couldn't sleep because my mind was racing thinking maybe, just maybe, things might improve.

July 31, 1990

So much for thinking things might be improving. Towards morning I was nauseous and ate a bit of fruit, as suggested by the chiropractor. Later, I took a bit of cereal and calcium and iron supplements. I felt very ill all that day. My feet were very swollen and red, I could barely walk. What the heck had I done to make me feel so bad again? The iron didn't seem to agree with me.

August 1, 1990

The summer is slipping by me again and I still have no concrete answers. Over 5 years, it seems impossible! What in the world was destroying me like this? I had another chiropractic treatment and I seemed to feel a bit better. It was expensive, but if it even helped a little it was worth it.

In the afternoon Rachelle and I sat in the sun and listened to music and talked. I feel fortunate that my children can share things with me and hope they can continue to do so. The sun felt good on my body and I started to daydream that we were on holidays in some exotic place, lying in the sun. I still tried to do positive imagery, as it was good therapy. In the evening we had company and I was able to visit. After they left Ken and I spent some special time together feeling very close and talking. These times were few and far between now. If I wasn't ill, then it was his colitis or we were just too stressed or exhausted. It seems that the evenings were better than mornings. I could not figure this out and obviously neither could anyone else.

That night I managed to sleep quite a few hours, even with getting up three times to go to the bathroom. Around 8:30 I got up and sat on the edge of the bed and felt very weak. I washed my face and hands and sat again on the edge of the bed thinking, I have to get to the kitchen and eat some fruit or something. I knew now that after eating in the morning, I seemed to feel a bit stronger.

I started walking to the kitchen and knew I was going to faint. I sat on the floor in the entrance to the kitchen by the pantry door; I could go no further. I reached up and opened the pantry door and looked at the cereal, raisins, crackers, etc. "Please God," I prayed, "help me, I can't even get to the phone." I couldn't stand to reach anything, so I grabbed the brown sugar, opened it and took some with my hand and put it in my mouth. I tried again to reach for some cereal, but it was too high. I sat there for about 2 minutes and suddenly I was amazed! I was able to get up and get a glass of water. Another few minutes and my head felt much better. I was still weak but no longer felt like fainting. "That must be it," I yelled out loud, "I must have diabetes or hypoglycemia." How in 5 years and all the tests I've had, could they miss something like that? I knew I was speculating but concluded it was okay to do so. Maybe, just maybe, speculating could lead to answers!

After eating breakfast I called my doctor's office and I was told to come in that afternoon. As I got ready to go, I tried to remember if anyone had done a glucose tolerance test on me and I didn't think they had. Lois picked me up to go to my appointment. I wondered how I could ever repay all her kindness.

My doctor did not seemed thrilled to see me, to say the least. I asked him if my iron test results were in because no one had called me. He said, "I'd tell you if there was something wrong." I then told him what had happened that morning and he looked at me as if I had completely lost it. Regardless, I went on and asked him if he felt I should have a glucose tolerance test. He said, "How could you take it? You have to fast and you might faint again." His sarcastic remark did little to provide the support I needed. I told him I would take the chance in the event it might provide some answers. I was booked for a glucose tolerance test for August 13.

When we got home, Lois asked me if I would mind if she took my blood sugar level with her son's diabetes kit. She took it after I had eaten and it was normal. She said she would come back before I ate the next morning and do it again. At 8:30 Lois came over and took my blood sugars and it was at the lower end of the normal range. It wasn't dangerously low. She gave me some juice and I felt a bit better and was able to make some breakfast.

I needed to wake up Rachelle so she could drive me to my chiropractor appointment. When would I ever be independent again? After my appointment we stopped at the hairdresser and treated Rachelle to a special haircut. As I watched, I thought how fortunate I was to have been blessed with such children. I thanked God for them and Ken and asked him to remember and help us so I wouldn't put these special people through this turmoil.

We decided to stop at Wendy's for a baked potato. I wasn't sure we should because I felt very weak, but didn't want to disappoint Rachelle. While she was getting lunch, I sat there and it was like I was there, but wasn't. People were talking and it was like they were far away. Rachelle was standing by me saying, "Mom, mom, are you okay? I think we should take this home." We stayed and ate a little but had to leave.

I lay on the sofa and stayed there. Rachelle asked if she could go horseback riding at a friend's. I asked her if her friend could possibly come over to our place instead, so I would have access to her if necessary.

I felt so ill and scared. A friend had given me the name of another internal specialist saying, "Please, please call him, you need another opinion." I called but was told I needed a referral. I desperately needed to talk to someone, anyone who could give me sound medical advice.

I called the lupus specialist I had seen at the Humanity Hospital but he wasn't in. I felt so sick and my throat and the front of my neck area hurt. I had no doubt the anxiety was making me worse. I decided to call my retired gynecologist. After all, he had known me for years. He also was unavailable.

Rachelle and I managed to make a little supper. After supper Ken said, "Come for a drive, it will do you good." I went with him but had to stay in the car when he went into the store. Now we all know that a woman has to be ill if she is unable to go into a shop! We came home and looked at the plans for a deck. A deck that we couldn't afford to build because of all this "crap" that was happening to us. I was exhausted and fell asleep instantly, only to awaken a few hours later with a weird sensation, like nothing in my body was functioning properly. I sat up most of the night and went back to sleep towards morning.

August 4, 1990

It's my Mother's birthday, and Robert's and Lorena's anniversary. I feel too ill to celebrate anything. Mom is at my sister Michelle's in Calgary for the summer holidays. It's just as well that she's away from all of this for a while. Janet, a friend from work, called and lifted my spirits up. Thank God for such people. I had a toast and re-read the article in Woman's Day about chronic fatigue syndrome (myalgic encephalomyelitis). Some of the symptoms I was experiencing were the same as in the article! It was a new name in medical terminology and many doctors were not interested or did not believe in this disease. Most likely because it was hard to diagnose and could mimic many other diseases. I decided to write to get more information on this disease.

I fell asleep that afternoon and awoke with my heart racing and my left hand numb. It was pretty scary, but by now I was quite reassured that I would survive all these strange things that were happening to my body. Had I not survived for over 5 years?

We made supper and I went outside with Ken. He was chopping wood and I felt a need to pull weeds or to do something. I sat on the edge of the garden for about 15 minutes and pulled a few weeds. I went into the house to wash my hands and had severe pain in my chest and felt very weak. I went back out and sat by the fire with Ken. After a while he asked if I wanted to go to the hardware store with him. I told him I would go because I was too afraid to stay alone. He gave me a funny look, and said, "The specialists are saying there is nothing wrong with you." How I hurt inside! I sat alone by the fire, furious at God for what was happening. Thank goodness that he loves unconditionally! Where were my children? I needed them so much. I knew I couldn't call them; everyone had had enough!

I hurt all over: my abdomen, stomach, my sides, my back, my arms and my neck. I have a terrible headache and my skin is so itchy. I'm weak and my feet burn and are swollen. All this and I'm not ill? Am I imagining this? I close my eyes and pray to die. Then I'm sorry for wishing it and try and convince myself that I have to keep going on.

August 7, 1990

Yesterday I had another appointment with the chiropractor. She reminded me I wasn't trying hard enough psychologically to get well. How little she knew about me! I had hardly slept again and the thought that I had to go through another test didn't help matters.

Rachelle drove me to the Sisters of Charity Hospital for a stomach test. I had called the hospital a few days earlier telling them I couldn't stand the pain any longer. They had called back telling me that the gastroenterologist had booked me earlier. I told Rachelle to go to the mall for a while. There was no way I would make her sit and wait in a hospital again. She had enough to handle on a daily basis and didn't need to hang around here. I had waited and gone through many tests alone and this one would be no exception. They did the gastroscopy and gave me two bags of Zantac intravenously. The doctor asked me why I hadn't spoken to my general practitioner about this problem because my stomach was very bad. I told her I had a number of times. She ordered blood work and gave me two prescriptions—Pepcid and Stelabid. The Zantac helped the burning in my stomach and when I got home I slept, and slept, as I had been given Demerol in the hospital.

On August 9 I called my doctor to see if they had the iron test results back. I was told he would call later but he didn't. At times I felt he wished I would vanish so he would not have to deal with me. I was becoming more of a thorn in his side than anything else.

I went to see the chiropractor. She asked me why I was getting a glucose tolerance test. She said, "We know your sugars are fine; don't do it to your body." She told me, "I had one foot in one camp and the other in another." She continued, "You'll have to decide which way you want to go." I explained to her that holistic medicine was still very new to me and I needed an adjustment period. She then asked me if I had been getting better or worse in the last 5 years. She definitely had a point there. At this time I felt I needed both opinions. I had to admit she was helping me cope and encouraged me to think positive.

August 10, 1990

I slept fairly well last night and feel a bit stronger. My sister Michelle called me in the evening and gave me the name of a book by Dr. Bernie Siegel. I had read of him and thought him to be a doctor who surpassed expectations in the impersonal world of medicine today. He is an ideal model of human caring for medical professionals.

On Saturday the 11th I worked in the garden on and off for a little while; then sat in the sun to see if it might help me. We had plans to go to a dinner theater with Linda and John that evening. I couldn't even remember when we had last attended a social function like this. I decided I would go and make the best of it. The worst that could happen was that I would have to come home. Ken was looking forward to this evening so much. I thought of all the evenings I had danced the night away not so long ago. Dancing was a love of mine. How I missed all those things.

Choosing a dress was a rude awakening. I always felt bloated and was sure I had gained weight because of the inactivity. I looked at my high-heeled shoes and decided I would try and wear some. It seemed impossible that 6 years ago I used to wear very high heels on a daily basis. When I put them on I realized how weak I really was. I was shaky as I walked to the dinner table, but with full make-up and my heels, I was determined to enjoy this evening. By the time we were seated, I felt that distant feeling and light-headedness so familiar to me. Once we ate I felt a bit better. We enjoyed the comedy and had some good laughs. My feet were burning and swelling and I had pain, but I was so glad for the company and laughter. Ken seemed so happy and I was able to stay the whole evening.

The next day we went to visit my father's grave. All the wonderful things about this special man came flooding back to me. Things like his patience, kindness and love of God. He was always so gentle and helpful to my mother and I would often hear him say, "Let me do that for you Mon Chou," which is a word of endearment in French, but in English means "my little cabbage." I could see him fixing the Christmas turkey and talking to it like he so often did and making us laugh. I asked him to help me and to share some of his strength. I so needed help and direction. I felt a warmth and calmness come over me and knew he was listening. I felt he was with me and saying, as he had so often done, "God loves you and is always with you. Trust in him." I was clearly given a sign that I had to reaffirm my faith and keep going. I had a strong feeling again that somehow I had to help others through my experience. How would I do this? At that time I really had no idea. I was well enough that evening to go to mass. I missed being in the choir. I loved to pray through song.

August 13, 1990

I had my glucose tolerance test and I felt incredibly weak since I couldn't eat or drink anything before the test. We discussed what was happening since I had been on the Zantac and medication prescribed by the gastroentologist. I told him my stomach felt somewhat well but my joints were worse. I had inflammation in the inner arms, inside my elbows, behind my knees and showed him how swollen my ankles were. The head noises were worse. I told him I lay out in the sun and wondered if that might make me worse. Also, I was now off Orudis. He just sat back, looked bewildered and let me talk.

I told him that I was considering going to a Chronic Fatigue Syndrome Clinic in the United States. He told me it was entirely up to me but it would be very expensive. I told him if I had his consent in writing, there would be a chance I might get financial assistance from Alberta Health Care. I continued that I needed answers for myself, my family, my employer and that I had to keep looking for answers if I was to try and get help.

I asked him if he felt we had covered everything like thyroid, liver, pancreas, etc. He said, "Yes that he had." We agreed we would wait until the glucose test results were in and until he got more information from my gastroscopy before I would make such a decision.

August 15, 1990

Rachelle must now feel like a taxi driver. Today is my appointment with the gastroenterologist to discuss my test results. She told me my stomach was very acidic and ulcerative. I told her the Zantac she had given me intravenously had helped with the burning. I asked her if the medication I was on could make my eyes dry and sore, but she kept on writing and ignored my question. I was told to take the Pepcid and Stelabid for 3 months. I told her I still felt very weak and like fainting. Did she think B12 shots might help? She said, "They really can't hurt you, I'll suggest it to your doctor and don't take the Orudis (anti-inflammatory) for 3 months." As I started to ask my next question, she was walking out the door. I said "Excuse me, I have another question. Has my liver been checked?" She replied that it had been done. I wondered why I had not been told this. I started asking another question, about possible absorption problems, but she was gone when I looked up. I sat there thinking she was attending to something and would return, but she didn't. I concluded my 7 minutes were up and that is all I would get. I couldn't help laughing and said to myself, "I could make a fortune giving communication seminars to the medical profession." I decided I could never be a doctor because I'd be broke talking to my patients at length. I left thinking the news wasn't so bad. An ulcerative and inflamed stomach; I could work at trying to cure that.

It doesn't seem possible that it's the middle of August. I have learned that by eating every 3 hours I don't feel like fainting. If I'm not careful I'll have a serious weight problem to deal with as well. Now, I can function a bit better with the fire put out in my stomach, but I still have very sore muscles, ringing and pulsating in the left ear and it is now starting in the right ear. I get so weak, tired and dizzy.

On August 16 I went back to the chiropractor. I still had problems accepting all the neck cracking, but once she had given me the "once over," I had to agree I did feel a bit better. I had my snack in the car and we stopped at my Mother's. She said her friends and her had been praying for me and surely God would help. I assured her he was listening and had a reason for all this. That night we all went out to eat for her birthday. It was late by the time they served supper and I was so light-headed I thought I would faint right there in the restaurant. I didn't say anything; I was not about to bring attention to me. I can't even say how many times I had to do this in front of family and friends. Finally the meal came. I had some chicken, vegetables and a potato. At 3 a.m. I was still trying to digest my meal. I could no longer eat a regular meal.

On August 17 I went to my doctor for a B12 shot and hoping for a miracle. He looked at my glucose tolerance test results quickly and said, "I think everything looks pretty normal here." I said, "Why is it I can't seem to go much more than 3 hours without feeling like I'm going to faint? That sounds like hypoglycemia to me, are you sure there's no indication of it on the test results?" He looked at the report again taking a little more time and turned the page over. "Oh yes, it does dip considerably after 3 hours. I guess that is indicative of hypoglycemia."

I was stunned! If I hadn't questioned him, he would not have looked at the test results again properly. How incredible! How much of this was going on? This was my doctor. I had put my trust in him. He gave me my B12 shot and looked at the insurance report he had to fill out. He said, "They want a full report and that will take time. Look at this file of yours." I told him someone would be back to pick it up. My total time with him that day was 12 minutes.

That evening I did not feel too bad. I imagined it would take more than one B12 shot to make a difference. I got a headache and my thighs felt like they were being blown up with air. By this time nothing that happened to my body surprised me. I assumed some of this was from the B12 shot.

August 18, 1990

My sister Terry called again. I know she can relate because she has been ill also. During her Florida holiday, she went to see a specialist at a "hard-to-diagnose" clinic. She said the doctor talked to her at great length about both of us and didn't even charge her. From the description of my symptoms he concluded I probably had hypoglycemia coupled with something else. If so, how could something like this have been missed? I had mentioned this at least four to five times over the last 5 years. At least we might have answers to one symptom.

Today was another bad day. I'm still congested and feel like I'm lacking air. My throat is sore and my chest feels tight. I tried vacuuming and had to stop and rest a lot. I feel like hell! So much for my miraculous cure!

I phoned my doctor to ask him to include that I wasn't sure if, or when, I could return to work. I felt like a child when he answered, "Now don't worry, I'll write the report to your insurance company." I replied, "I know you will, I just wanted to clarify a few things." I also asked him if an appointment could be made with a specialist so I could get direction regarding the hypoglycemia findings. He said, "Make an appointment and we'll set it all up when you come in." This was getting ridiculous. Why would I have to see him so they could phone a specialist? There was absolutely no need for him to see me again for that.

I went to bed with a small glass of milk and half a banana by my bed. I found that if I ate a bit around 4 a.m. that I didn't feel like fainting when I got up.

August 19, 1990

I had a better sleep last night. I'm so grateful for the nights that provide me with the rest I so desperately need and the escape from the nightmare in our lives. I had my snack at 5 a.m. and got up at 8 a.m. My thighs and leg muscles are twitching badly today and I have a lot of zinging in my head. Today I'm having trouble writing and I find that most frightening. What is wrong with me? Is it neurological? But so many doctors have examined me.

The children came over today and we went out for pizza with Bernie, May and their children. Although company tired me, I loved the distraction. These people are constant reminders that I have to "hang in there" and keep looking for help. In the evening the children went for horseback rides and we sat around the fire.

On Monday I called the lupus specialist at the Humanity Hospital. He spoke to me at length and seems like an incredible human being. He had seen me once and was willing to talk to me on the phone whenever I called. He finished by saying, "I'm very interested in your case, please call me and let me know what happens. I think you should see an endocrinologist as soon as possible. Good luck, I'll be thinking of you Annette." Immediately after I hung up, I called my general practitioner's office and asked if they could please make a referral to the Humanity Hospital Endocrinology Clinic on an emergency basis. I explained my last conversation with my general practitioner and said I felt I shouldn't have to go in to get a referral. They assured me they would speak to the doctor and get back to me as soon as possible.

At this time I'm still taking the medication prescribed by the gastroentologist. I was taking 1000 mg of calcium, as the holistic chiropractor had suggested, but had to cut it down to 500 mg because my stomach was bothering me.

My doctor's office returned the call a few hours later telling me the doctor wants me to see him so that we can discuss the referral. Another appointment was booked for Wednesday at 5:30 p.m. What an abuse of the medical system I thought. How many doctors were doing this?

I picked a few vegetables from the garden. How I long for my lost energy as I sit and rest after only a few minutes work. How we take things for granted and forget to thank God for the gift of good health.

My left side seems to be hurting me much more lately, so I'm trying to eat very small portions at a time. I have canceled the chiropractic appointment this week, as it's getting too expensive. I still have not received any money from my insurance company.

My sister Michelle sent us a movie called "Leap of Faith." It is a true story about a woman with cancer and how she was healed with the help of positive imagery, acupuncture, herbs and changing her eating habits. How we related to this couple as we watched. It was an excellent film and provided us with incentive to keep going and to keep searching for answers.

As I look back, I now realize it must have been sheer determination to survive that kept me from giving up completely. I would look at my husband and children and say, "I don't want to die, I want to live to see my children and grandchildren get married." I continued to tell myself that one day I would walk, bike, garden and even dance again. "I will sing a song all the way through without feeling out of breath and too tired to finish it," I said.

As I sat on the porch that night I thanked God for the strength he gave me each day to cope. I asked his forgiveness for the times I despaired and prayed one day he would touch me with his kindness and heal me. Alone that night, I felt a shiver run through me, then, I felt warm as if someone had covered me with a blanket. I knew again that

God had heard me and as I got up to go inside I prayed, "Please God, show me the way."

August 21, 1990

As I write in my diary, I see the first light of dawn. Another day and I'll keep fighting this illness. At about 4 a.m. I had a small piece of banana. I'm at a point where I don't know what to eat, but I do know that if I eat something sweet I don't feel like fainting. I am anxious to see the endocrinologist and get some direction in regards to my hypoglycemia. The young lupus specialist had explained to me that glucose was a hormone and a body could not function properly without it. I hoped that the things that had happened to my body could be reversed enough to let me improve the quality of my life and the life of others around me. At 6 a.m. I had a digestive cookie and went back to bed to see if I could get a little sleep. I fell asleep instantly but woke up not long after and felt far away, like I was awake, but wasn't. My left hand was numb and I had trouble getting up. I could barely get to the kitchen. Why did this happen? I ate a toast with a little peanut butter but felt the same. At 10 a.m. I ate a chocolate bar and felt somewhat better but it only lasted an hour. I then ate some soup and a piece of cheese. It seemed like I was now spending my days eating and wondering when and what I should eat to see if I might feel better.

My legs look swollen and my arms hurt so much. I'm alone and I momentarily loose it. I yell, "Damn, I'm probably going to die of overeating now. What am I doing this for?" I scream and yell over and over, "Someone help me, please, I don't know what I'm doing. Help me, help me." I fall to the floor close to hysteria and scream and sob. I don't know how long I sat there on the floor; but I remember slowly getting up and saying, "What are you doing now, how can you do this after promising yourself to think positive and not lose it like this?" I talk myself up again.

Rachelle and Ken are gone to a horse-jumping clinic. For the rest of the day I watched television and that was the extent of it. It had been a long hard day and I would try to make tomorrow a better day.

August 22, 1990

I'm not feeling very well today, but it's better than yesterday. I went outside and picked a few vegetables while sitting on a pail turned upside-down. I'm very weak and light-headed, but have decided I have to accomplish something daily regardless how I feel. I had, in the past, accomplished things by setting goals for myself and wanted to continue to establish daily goals no matter how small. This was very important to me psychologically.

We decided to do a few errands in town before our 5:30 appointment with the doctor. Ken saw a hobby shop and thought it might please me to go in for a while. No sooner were we in the door that I had to ask for a chair and couldn't even look around. I looked at the women talking and walking all over the store and wondered how they did it. I was so very tired and weak; I could have laid down right there on the floor.

When we got to the doctor's office he seemed surprised that I had asked for a referral to the Humanity Hospital Endocrinology Department. I explained again that it had been highly recommended. Since hypoglycemia had been detected, an appointment with such a specialist might just make life a little better for us. He looked at me and said, "Don't you trust my judgment?" I told him I did, but felt at this point in time that we should work together with any specialist who might give us answers and direction. I reminded him that I had a job that I would love to go back to as soon as possible and the school term was beginning in another week.

I knew deep inside that I would not be able to go back this term or, at least, not at the beginning of it. I asked him to inform my insurance company that I would go back to work when I could cope with it and when I got help and dietary direction. He seemed again surprised at my assertiveness and let me speak without interruption. As I looked at him I felt sorry for him again, he looked so confused about it all. He reminded me that a lot of my symptoms did not point to hypoglycemia. We discussed this and concluded it was a place to start anyway.

After our talk he said he would send a referral letter to the Humanity Hospital, if that was what I wanted. He asked me if I had brought my B12 with me and I reminded him that I had my first shot only 5 days before. We discussed this and he concluded it might be too soon to tell if it would help and too soon for another B12 shot.

I sit in our cozy living room with the fireplace on and look at the quiet rain outside. I work on my positive imagery. Rain rarely depresses me; I always feel at peace when I watch the earth and trees drink the water. I looked out at our horse Angel; she will foal in the spring and hoped things would go well for her. I think of Rachelle who will be starting Grade 11. It seems impossible.

August 24, 1990

I called my doctor's office to see if the appointment had been made for me at the Metabolic Centre. I was informed that the appointment had been made for 7:30 a.m. on the 28th and that I had to fast. After lunch Rachelle and I went to get a few groceries. At first I was managing quite well, but after about half an hour I could have laid down in the isle by the vegetables and simply slept.

In addition to our current problems, Ken was now concerned about cutbacks at work in the spring. In the evening we went for a drive and stopped at A&W for a Root Beer. I was always wondering now if I should be eating or drinking such things. Being there brought memories back of times gone-by when it was the thing to do. We tried not to talk about all the nightmarish things we were dealing with and talked about positive things. We agreed it was the only way we would make it through this.

Saturday, August 25, 1990

I slept quite well last night. I took a Pepcid before my night snack and it seemed to help my stomach. I took milk during the night as suggested by the dietitian on the phone. It seemed to hold me better than a piece of fruit but made me feel very bloated.

Rachelle and Ken have left for another horse show. How I wish I could help more with these things and be there all day like most of the other moms. Ken will come back and pick me up later. It was cold and damp at the horse show, which wasn't the best thing for my inflammation and joints. Rachelle was great and won 6 first-places. She is getting to be an incredible little rider. I had to close my eyes when she went over the last few jumps; they seemed so high and difficult. She laughed and said, "Mom, why do you come to watch me and close your eyes at the best time?"

August 27, 1990

Today I had my appointment with the specialist-in-charge of cardiology at the Sisters of Charity Hospital. I confirmed the appointment twice. I wasn't about to be told I didn't have the right time again. He was not convinced I had hypoglycemia, but possibly a lupus-type disease that might cause the symptoms. He agreed it was systematic and it caused a lot of inflammation and all kinds of other symptoms. He told me a disease such as lupus could cause fluid around the heart. He said he would check to make sure the test results were indeed a false positive. I was amazed this had not already been done! He ordered another 24 hour Holter tape to see if there was a heart beat change. I informed him I would send him the test result information from the Humanity Hospital in the event it might help him with a diagnosis.

Back home I tried to do a little ironing but had to stop, as the inflammation was so bad. I couldn't take Orudis for the inflammation so I took coated Aspirin and that helped a bit. I sat there trying to figure out what all the doctors had said and what I should do to follow up on this lupus thing that everyone seemed to be bringing up. Had I not already seen specialist in regard to this? Tomorrow I had to go to the Metabolic Centre. How could I keep everything straight with so many doctors?

August 28, 1990

Rachelle, my little driver, took me to my 7:30 a.m. appointment. The doctor was very business-like and seemed thorough. He asked a lot of questions regarding the questionnaire I had just completed. I was very light-headed and had trouble concentrating and answering all the questions. He examined me and said he would look at my concerns from the hypoglycemia point of view. I had to go for blood work again. I feel like a pincushion! As I left, I asked him to please sent the results to my doctor as soon as possible.

We had toast at the hospital cafeteria. I told Rachelle to go register for school and that I would walk the 3 blocks to the ENT specialist where she could pick me up. That was not too smart on my part. The 3 blocks seemed like 3 miles and I was totally exhausted by the time I got there. He checked my hearing and said it didn't seem to have changed since the last time he saw me in 1988. I told him about how my neck, ear and side of the face hurt. He looked at my throat and said I had what looked like viral ulcers and that could cause the sore throat. I asked him why I had these most of the time and he answered, "Have you been checked for lupus?" Everyone thought I had lupus, except the lupus specialists. I was so tired when I got back home that I stayed in bed the rest of the afternoon. How I was tired, tired, tired of going to doctors.

Lorena came over with Daniel for a few hours this week. It was so nice to have some time with them, what a lovely distraction. We picked a few vegetables from the garden for them. Ken and I cut some borders from wallpaper for our bedroom. I couldn't work long periods because of the cramping in my hands.

My department superintendent called and asked if I knew someone who might want to replace me for a few months or more. I gave him a few names and was concerned about them finding someone for September. He was very kind and reassuring about my job and hopes I'll be back when I can and reminded me they missed me. I told him I missed everyone and my work as well.

August 30, 1990

I did a little housework in the morning and seem to have a little more strength, but the inflammation is much worse. I went to see the psychiatrist and brought him up-to-date on what had happened over the last month. He asked me what medication I was taking and I told him Pepcid and Stelabid. He told me the side effects of Stelabid could be dangerous and to stop taking it immediately. He said, "I don't know why gastroentologists prescribe this medication. Continue the Pepcid and stop the other now." I told him I was suffering from bad stomach problems and felt like fainting, especially in the mornings. He explained how our brain cells are mainly made of glucose and how important it was that hypoglycemia is controlled properly. He added this disease could cause depression also.

I then made an appointment with my general practitioner. A young Chinese intern saw me first and when my doctor came in I told them who I had recently seen and what they had said. The doctor said he thought I looked a bit better than when I last saw him. I told him I was trying to control my diet and I seemed to be feeling a bit stronger. I showed them my hands and feet and asked again about the inflammation. He told me I could try Orudis again and continue taking the Pepcid with another antacid. When I asked about the dietitian, he said, "Don't you remember we got you one?" I answered that the dietitian he was referring to was the one in the hospital who provided me with a diet plan because my jaws were so sore. He told me he would see what the doctor from the Metabolic Centre would say first. He told me he would give me another B12 shot but the intern said, "I think you should give her only one a month." He agreed and decided to wait for another 2 weeks. Before I left, I asked him to please call me when he received results from any of the doctors I had recently seen. I was so tired when I got home that I went to bed. My body and brain just could no longer function.

On August 31 I had trouble emotionally dealing with the fact that my peers were going back to work and I couldn't be there. The psychiatrist had reminded me that I had been ill for a long time and it would take a long time to get better. He told me progress might be very slow when I began to improve. I called my insurance company again.

September 1, 1990

Another month has passed. Will this be a better one? Things simply had to improve. Ken had a bad colitis attack this morning. Now his stress level is up because of the cutbacks at work. I do hope we don't lose our home; we love it here and have worked so hard to get to this point. Ken and Rachelle have left for a 3-day horse show. Ken will come back on Monday and bring me to the stadium show.

These are the times when it is so hard to be this incapacitated. Times when I want to help my children or attend
functions with them. My long-term goal for the summer was
to clean my kitchen cupboards, something I used to do in a
weekend. Now it was a shelf at a time, if I could.

On Sunday I couldn't go to the horse show so I read
and rested. Mornings are still bad; I'm weak and light-
headed for long periods. I find it so hard to stay alone and
it gets very difficult to stay positive at times. I started on two
Orudis again for the inflammation. I can barely walk or
work with my hands for the pain. I'm torn, I know I'm not
supposed to take this medication for another 2 months because of my stomach, but I have to try and control the
inflammation in my body. I carry Tums around with me. I
didn't get the Diovol because it contained aluminum and I
felt I didn't need that in my body at this time.

On Monday I went to the horse show and enjoyed it. I
tried to walk a bit and my legs seemed to carry me a bit
better. I was so tired that night I fell asleep as soon as my
head hit the pillow, only to awaken with bad pain shortly
after.

September 4, 1990

Today is hard because Ken and Rachelle have left for
work and school. It's not that I dislike staying at home, it's
the reason that I have to stay home that I have trouble with.
I decided to rest and then try to do another shelf in my
cupboards. I couldn't do any cupboards today. Rachelle
came home at noon and we did a few errands together.

In the evening we went to celebrate Daniel's second
birthday. It's hard to believe he is already 2 years old. He's

talking so well for his age and we enjoy him enormously. At 8 p.m., while waiting for supper, I had to ask Lorena for a piece of cheese and a cracker because I was feeling so weak. We went for a short walk because I couldn't walk more than a few blocks. I get so embarrassed and frustrated when this happens.

That night I didn't sleep well and when I did, I had nightmares. I dreamt I was seeing a doctor for the pain in my head and he was trying to figure out what was causing the pulsating, ringing and zinging. I was strapped to a table and he was standing by me naked from the waist up. I'm glad it wasn't from the waist down! He took pictures of my head and kept saying he would heal me. When he met me in his office, he was in a blue-stripped suit, took me by the hand and brought me out of the building. He left me there alone and I was lost and frightened and sick. I was crying when Ken woke me up. He held me and told me it was only a nightmare and that everything would be fine. I was so glad for the comfort of his arms. I desperately needed it and at times was so afraid to tell him how I felt or that he would see me cry.

Last night I heard on the news that chronic fatigue syndrome was often misdiagnosed and people are being called psychosomatic amongst other things. They continued to say that the mislabeling increased their problems. I, for one, fully understand this. Apparently research was being done to see if it is viral or contagious. As I listened to this, I wondered if I could have this new and misunderstood disease. After all the specialists I had seen, surely it would have been discovered; or, was it so new that no one understood what it was? If nothing happened this month, I decided I would gather any test results that I could and go to the Chronic Fatigue Syndrome Clinic in the United States. We would have to approach Alberta Health Care for financial assistance. I still had not heard from my insurance company. I decided to call Toronto again, of course, at my expense. The insurance company informs me my file has gone to the medical director for approval and I should hear from them soon. How many times had I heard that story?

It has been a week since I've been to the Metabolic Centre and have no results yet. I can't believe no one is helping me with a proper diet plan. My neighbor down the road invited me for tea this afternoon and I decided to go. It was the furthest I had walked for a long time, about 3 or 4 blocks. When I got there I was shaking and had to stop numerous times on the way there, but I had made it. I was craving company so much and the possibility that I might feel anything like normal that I would have most likely crawled there. I would never admit to them that I couldn't walk there. It was a nice hour and I did accept a ride to go back home with a neighbor who had to pass by our house. That evening Terry called again and we talked about the new findings regarding chronic fatigue syndrome. She felt I should look into this further, as soon as possible.

The next morning I called the Chronic Fatigue and Immunology Deficiency Syndrome Organization in Portland, Oregon. I talked to a man named Bill who was very nice and said he had heard of many people who were told they were hypochondriacs, etc. He said he would send me information, as well as, information for my doctor. I called the young lupus specialist who was as interested and as nice as ever. He told me an infectious disease specialist at the Humanity Hospital was interested in this new and alarming disease. When he told me his name I remembered I had seen him in 1986. He was one of the doctors that suspected heart trouble. He was a good doctor and no doubt he would be most interested because it was within his area of work. I decided to make an appointment with this doctor.

In the morning I decided to weigh myself and was shocked to see how much weight I had gained. I decided I had to lose 30 to 40 pounds. I had never been this heavy, but what could I expect when I was eating every 2 to 3 hours. My portions were not large but I had to cut these down even more. I walked around the yard a bit and decided I had to push myself to the limit.

On Saturday Ken and I decided we should go for a drive to a little town near our city. We then thought that maybe it wasn't such a good idea as we were so financially strapped that month. What a nightmare, we were really looking forward to getting out for a drive. It seemed like all I did was go to doctors. How I wished I would never have to see another one. I'm so congested this morning and I try doing some deep breathing to see if it will help. My throat is still sore all the time. "Dear God, help me keep sane through this. Take me by the hand. I need your help," I pray.

Ken had to go back to bed for a while because of a colitis attack last night. In the afternoon we decide to go for a drive anyway. I tried walking up and down Main Street but had to come back to the car because I was so weak and my legs and feet were so sore. We spent $50 that day we couldn't really afford, but were glad we had gone. The distraction had been good therapy for us. What in the world was that insurance company waiting for anyway.

September 9, 1990

Last night I had a nightmare about our finances. It was terrible! Trucks were coming into our yard and the men were all dressed in white. They were laughing and moving our furniture out, even our heirlooms. Our house was bare and someone was hammering a big "For Sale" sign to our fence. Ken woke me up and asked if I had been dreaming. I told him I had, but not what it was about. My legs are very swollen this morning and I feel bloated. I have to keep going for fear that if I stop, I'll stop for good.

I went outside with Ken and sat on the ground to try and help with the weeds. My arms and legs got very sore, but I was mad and kept pulling and crying. This thing was not going to get me! I refused to let it completely consume me! We went to church in the evening and there were times I got so annoyed at God for not giving us answers and help. Yet by the end of mass, I had gained strength to carry on in whatever way I could.

On Monday the 10th I called my insurance company again and this is the message I got. "The news is not too good," he said, "Your doctor's report didn't indicate it was imaginary and that you could go to work, but it didn't say you couldn't." I was deeply hurt that the doctor, who had seen me suffer so much and whom I had put my confidence in, had not supported me. Had I wasted all my time thinking he was really concerned and trying to help me? I just blew up at the insurance representative. All the frustration and hurt poured out. I was usually good at controlling my emotions, but I let him have it with both barrels. I told him, as my contact, he should be fighting for my case. Did he not believe how ill I was? I told him they would be receiving a letter from me.

I sat down and started to write, what was to become a 22-page letter, to the insurance company. I included documentation from my daily diary as to what was happening to me. Because I had trouble writing, it took me 3 days to write the letter that would finally shed light on my situation. I informed them I would see a doctor of their choice. They answered that a nurse would be sent to see me. I wondered what that would accomplish after all the specialists I had seen. I then called my doctor's office and asked them for a copy of the report sent to the insurance company. I asked them to have it ready for me to pick up on Thursday when I went in for my next appointment. About 15 minutes later, the doctor himself called saying we would discuss this request on Thursday. I told him I needed a copy because I wanted to see a lawyer about the insurance company delaying my payments. It is my understanding that it is legal to obtain copies of our medical files, test results reports, etc.

I was very ill that afternoon and the added stress had not helped. My legs felt like the skin would burst. Was it inflammation or fluid? You would think the medical doctors could at least tell me that! I get tired at times of researching to try to find answers. The appointment with the Infectious Disease specialist is not until November 11, more than 2 months away. I wonder if I should go to the specialist in Calgary. He, however, had told me by phone he felt it wasn't lupus. I sat on the porch, waiting for Rachelle to return from her horseback ride, and prayed, "Please Lord, don't let us lose our home because we can't collect from my insurance company." What has happened to our society when we can't collect insurance after paying for so long in the event something like this should happen?

September 11, 1990

I woke up in the middle of the night with severe vertigo and like something was moving in my head. I hate it when this happens because I wake up screaming and startle Ken. He holds me and tells me it will be okay. I so appreciate his kindness through this nightmare. There has to be something causing this "seizure-type" thing, but what? This morning I have a lot of involuntary movement in my left hand and inflammation and redness in my body. Because of my stomach, I had to stop taking the Orudis and calcium. I'm still taking Pepcid and Tums in hopes something will help. My friend Debbie called and asked if I had called her doctor yet for another opinion. I told her I had and he was not taking new patients at this time.

Lois came over and said she had spoken to her dietitian and had asked her to call me. She called me shortly after and gave me some direction on what to eat. She told me she would make an appointment and have someone call me regarding the time. We can't believe how long it is taking to get results from the Metabolic Centre and diet help.

On Thursday we went to my general practitioner. After waiting an hour he gave me his report to my insurance company to read. It was five pages of notes, quite in a mumble jumble. Things were not clarified, not correct or there was missing information. I asked for a copy, but he refused saying the insurance company had requested it and they would have to give him permission to released a copy to me. I told him I was surprised at this, after all, was it not regarding my medical condition?

I discussed the chronic fatigue thing with him again and told him my sister Terry had called Dr. French in Montreal who was heading the Canadian research on this new disease. He told me I had made the right choice by calling the infectious disease specialist regarding this. He said, "One out of three of my patients complain of fatigue." I answered that if the percentage was that high, that as a physician, I would be very concerned. He again said it was difficult to diagnose as it mimicked so many other diseases. Before I left he gave me another B12 shot in the event it might help.

I called the infectious disease specialist's office to see if I could get in sooner. I was told the date I was given would be the soonest that he could see me. I told her I had called Dr. French in Montreal and he had suggested I get in to see this specialist as soon as possible. The young lady hesitated and, after a few minutes, said she could book me for October 17. I guess a month wait was better than two.

September 14, 1990

Another bad night! I woke up around 3 a.m. with a lot of head noises. When I went back to sleep I had more nightmares. Someone was trying to saw my head in half and telling me it was time to replace the bad half. He then brought me into this other room where all these half heads were lined on a shelf, but none matched my face. They were all the same and looked like plastic. I woke up crying and soaking wet. Why was I having such terrible night-mares? It was a bad day again. My legs were swollen and very sore, but I went for my short walk anyway.

I called the insurance company again to get permission to copy the report from the doctor. He said I would have to get a lawyer to request this. Get a lawyer when we couldn't afford one because they were keeping money from me that was rightfully mine. He said he would speak to his manager and that he would send me one cheque for now. I couldn't understand the logic of this. Why were they stalling so much? What kind of proof did they need that I was sick? I told him about the two doctors who were interested in chronic fatigue syndrome and that I was following this up. He asked me to repeat this so he could write it down. I reminded him that this insurance problem was not helping. I lay down exhausted. Along with the other symptoms I was now getting a bad rash.

On Saturday, while Ken and Rachelle went to a horse show, I stayed with Lorena, Robert and Daniel. I went for a little walk with Daniel. In the afternoon I slept and had nightmares. I felt weak and tired and my legs were sore all day. Ken and I had supper there and we left early because I was so tired. How I long for good health, it is everything. What a shame our government doesn't promote preventive medicine in the form of more information to the public about diet and the importance of physical activity. Health programs in the work place might reduce a lot of time off for sickness. Why are things like physical education and health courses considered less important in schools? Why are underground garages permitted in public work places and shopping centres? Etc., etc., etc.

On Sunday I felt a little bit better. I had no idea why some days I could at least function and other days I was basically bedridden and could barely walk. The better days were far and few between, but how I was grateful for them. We went grocery shopping and again the lights bothered me. Ken is having difficulty today with our financial situation and I feel to blame for it. Again I'm annoyed that the doctor hadn't supported us in his report to the insurance company. Also, that the insurance company can't do what it promises to do. I have stopped drinking milk and feel less bloated. I also want to see if the congestion improves.

On the 17th I received a call from the Diet Centre at the Humanity Hospital. I was given an appointment for the 28th (my birthday). I am anxious to get more direction regarding diet. I called my secretary at work to see how things were going. The lady replacing me was over and we went over a lot of the duties in that position. I do miss being there and hope all the deadlines will be met.

Lois called and told me about a lady in the subdivision named Gerda who had been diagnosed as having chronic fatigue syndrome. She gave me her phone number and suggested I call her. I called her and she came right over. We talked and cried together. She has been ill for 2 years, compared to my 6. She understood what I was going through. She gave me Dr. Dare's name and number and told me to call right away. She explained that he was a naturopathic M.D. I felt the two types of doctor degrees had to be impressive! I thanked her for her support and help and told her I would let her know what he said. Gerda is a wonderful person and we have since become friends with her and her husband Ed. I called and Dr. Dare answered himself and booked me for that Thursday, September 20, 1990. I needed a referral for Health Care purposes and I called my general practitioner's office and the receptionist said she could do that for me. My hopes were up. Maybe, just maybe, I would get help here!

Thursday, September 20, 1990

That morning Ken dropped me off at my Mother's before the appointment. She lived only about 2½ blocks from the doctor's office. I was very "puffy" that day and my feet burned and hurt. I decided I would walk there with Mom, thankful for her support.

We walked into a very plain office, there was no receptionist and I could hear the doctor talking to a woman and her young son. In the small waiting room, the husband and baby waited. Apprehensive to begin with, it was a relief to see someone else there. As I waited, I wondered why I was bothering with another doctor. Again, it would surely lead nowhere.

My apprehension was soon put to rest as this gentle and intelligent man talked and listened to me for 1½ hours. "Yes Annette," he said, "you are sane but a very sick lady." He felt I had something called Chronic Fatigue Immune Deficiency Syndrome. He explained that I had most likely come in contact with some toxins, might have Candida

Yeast Syndrome and there was probably a post-viral factor. I looked at him quite incredulous and tears began to fall.

He proceeded to explain in detail how this could happen. He lost me with his chemistry but he added he would explain how he would treat my disorder. I felt I had been handed a gift. Someone at last believed me and would try to help me. He explained to me in great detail what each "non-drug" supplement would do for me. We left with my papers of explanations and a heart full of hope! Later that evening I called Gerda and thanked her for giving me Dr. Dare's name.

Ken and I went and bought our bag full of hope and left a lot of money behind. Of course, Health Care does not recognize natural medicines. Why not? I don't understand. If it can help after trying everything else, then natural medicine should be included.

Monday, September 24, 1990

I had not started the new program on the weekend. I went to a horse show and wanted to make sure that I took the different pills at the right times.

Today I decided to start the program. As I lined up the bottles on the counter, I couldn't help but be a little frightened. Had I not been told by a practitioner that vitamins and mineral pills only gave a person expensive urine. I decided I would eat a pail of these right now if it would make me feel better. Anything... I would try anything!

My program consisted of acidophilus, evening primrose oil (an essential polyunsaturated fatty acid), Ester C (vitamin C), zinc, B6, kelp, CoQ10, vitamin A (cod liver oil), vitamin E, calcium, magnesium and a multivitamin with "everything in it." In addition, L-phenylalanine (an essential amino acid), flax oil (another essential fatty acid) and Nystatin to kill the candida yeast.

September 26, 1990

This is my third day on the program. Already it seems like I don't feel so bloated and the pain in my legs seems to be less severe. The Nystatin is upsetting my stomach and I have some headaches. Like I was told, the "die off" of the yeast would cause this. I wonder if the constant pulsating and ringing in my left ear will eventually go. As Dr. Dare said, "You have been ill for a long time, it will take time for you to improve." I'm too impatient; I want it to work now!

Yesterday Gerda came over again. What a nice lady she is and I know that we will become friends. It is hard to believe that someone can really relate to this nightmare. She has been ill for 2 years and has four children. She feels Dr. Dare's program has helped her a lot and tells me she is also going to a massage therapist. I asked her to make me an appointment. After she leaves, I think I should have discussed this with Ken to see if we can afford it.

I have not returned to the holistic chiropractor. We simply can't afford her and she wanted me to go back twice a week. I still feel like a rubber ball, being tossed around to everyone. I hope this new program will help my memory. It's so frustrating.

Dr. Dare also gave me two books that he has written on yeast syndrome and I devour them. He is truly a devoted doctor who spends up to 2 hours with his patients. No wonder he can't afford a receptionist. Dr. Dare put me on a sugar-free diet and I'm keeping track of everything I eat.

Today I received a letter from Dr. Cord at the Metabolic Centre. He indicated my tests were normal and that he wanted to repeat a morning Cortisol test. Dr. Dare had explained how yeast syndrome could cause hypoglycemia. I certainly have some form of it.

Monday, October 15, 1990

I have now been on Dr. Dare's program for 3 weeks. The first week my stomach was upset, but he said the Nystatin could cause this. By the second week I felt a little stronger. The most apparent was the improvement of my mental capacities. My memory seemed better and my mind seemed "sharper." I didn't seem to feel so "spaced out." By the third week I was strong enough to drive into Sherwood Park. To me, it was a milestone. I even went to the garden and cut perennials for a while.

In the evening I thought I'd try a Jacuzzi. Well, it happened again. I felt worse after. The muscles in my legs, arms and neck were moving involuntarily. My eyes felt funny (like nerves jumping). The pulsating and ringing in my ears was much worse last night. It kept me awake for part of the night. My hands were red and puffy and I wondered if it was something that I had eaten. Was it the hot water, the Jacuzzi, or both? Did I have damaged nerves? I rested most of that morning.

As I was writing to my insurance company, I received a call from their representative telling me my claim for help had finally been approved. I thanked God for this as it was one less thing to worry about and I could concentrate on getting help and feeling better.

I called Dr. Benhar, a homeopathic doctor, to see if he could look at possible food intolerances. Dr. Dare knows this person so I feel better about seeing him. Apparently he works with a machine and sensor, which reads and graphs intolerances to foods, can indicate candida levels, and detect if there is something wrong with organs. This sounds quite incredible and should be very interesting.

I'm not loosing much weight and still feel "puffy," although not as much. I wonder if it's fluid or inflammation, maybe both. I'm going to Dr. Tell (infection specialist) on Wednesday. It will be interesting to see what he has to say.

October 22, 1990

Last Thursday I went to see Dr. Tell. He was with me for over an hour. I shared everything with him. I gave him a copy of the information sent to my insurance company, the Chronic Fatigue Syndrome information from Portland and blood test result information. I shared with him what the psychiatrist had said and the frustration experienced from all the labels pinned on me. He said, "One of our researchers had come down with this chronic fatigue syndrome." I imagined this had made him more sympathetic to my condition. He felt my rashes were due to food intolerance, allergies or environmental causes. He checked me and ordered a lot of blood work. He added it could be viral related. I am very anxious to get these results.

I made an appointment on Thursday for Ken and myself with Dr. Dare. I felt that he might be able to help Ken with his colitis.

October 23, 1990

The visit with Dr. Benhar was most interesting. According to him, my allergies were high, especially to chemicals, fungus and molds. Also, I had a very high intolerance to over 50 foods. I found him easy to talk with and a very positive person. His electrodiagnosis machine was called an "Interro." He prescribed homeopathic drops and said I should feel improvement in a week. These drops could be taken along with the supplements Dr. Dare had suggested. An appointment was made for a follow-up visit in a month.

That afternoon I had an appointment with a new dentist regarding a root canal problem. Going to a dentist has never been a joy for me, especially a new one. A number of x-rays were taken and he concluded the root canal was okay. He said I had problems in my left jaw joint and that could be causing the left ear discomfort. An appointment was made to have fillings replaced, to reduce some of the amalgam that might be toxic to my body. The toxic thing was really starting to make sense to us.

October 27, 1990

Ken is working on the barn and Rachelle is doing her homework. I look out at the countryside and thank God for helping me find some answers. I have a little less pain in my arms and legs and am feeling stronger. I realize it's not a huge improvement, but my spirits are lifted. My interest levels are up and life seems better in general.

I have been on Dr. Benhar's (homeopath) medication for allergies HS14 and HS23 relating to molds, chemicals, and foods, and numerous chemical intolerances. I have not eaten foods that he told me I had intolerances to. For the first 5 days I had a headache. I called him and he told me, "Hang in there. You are experiencing withdrawal symptoms and your body is adjusting. It will be gone before the end of the week." He was right; by Friday it had left me.

I continue to take Dr. Dare's natural medication as directed. Ken and I went to see him on the 25th. He is testing Ken for his colitis and for general fatigue. He has only been on Dr. Dare's program since yesterday so we are anxious to see if it will help his colitis, which is now worse.

The ringing and pulsating in my head and ears seems a bit better. I've noticed that it seems the worst between 2 a.m. and the time I get up. That is a definite mystery. It's thought it could be from my car accident. All in all, there is improvement and I'm in a very positive frame of mind.

November 7, 1990

I'm still on the programs of Drs. Dare and Benhar. Improvement is still happening. It is slow, but definitely there! I find the elimination of so many foods difficult, especially breads (no wheat products), pastas, etc. Yesterday I had a friend over and we cheated on my foods.

Today I'm not feeling quite so well. I'm very tired. I also had 5 fillings done on Monday, so that might be the reason.

I completed the Canada Pension form and I also sent the necessary information to the insurance company. There will be a rehabilitation person coming over. This is to check on me, no doubt. What a waste of money! My rehabilitation is following my current programs, resting, doing positive thinking, etc.

I am currently reading "Peace, Love and Healing" by Dr. Bernie Seigel. What an amazing human being he is with an attitude a lot of doctors could benefit from. Following his suggestions regarding imagery and visualization along with practicing positive thinking have helped me.

I've started driving a little and have done a bit of Christmas shopping. As I slowly walk into a store, I am in tears of joy. I hope I can go to work and say hello to everyone soon.

November 12, 1990

This week is starting off better. I'm feeling stronger and my arms don't hurt as much. My legs still bother me as well as the ringing and pulsating is still there. My brother Bernie sent me a book on reflexology. It sounds quite interesting. I had previously read about foot reflexology, but this incorporates the whole body.

November 19, 1990

This is not a good morning and I don't know what has gone wrong? I have a severe headache and I'm weak and my stomach is upset. I went with Ken to Rachelle's Provincial Volleyball Meet for 3 days. I probably got overtired and ate the wrong foods. It is not easy to eat in restaurants when having to eat only specific foods. I'll be anxious to see what Dr. Benhar's test results are on December 5.

I finally have an appointment with Drenda, a massage therapist. It will be interesting to see how I feel after this.

November 30, 1990

Yesterday I had my very first therapeutic massage. The room was downstairs and it took me awhile to get down because my joints were still bad. I was expecting the treatment to be more painful because of the inflammation in my body. The therapist said the first time she would work more gently and concentrate on my upper back and neck. She explained how this would help release the toxins from my body. I was warned I might feel worse after the first or second treatment. She was right; I felt good right after, but the next day the pulsating seemed worse. I was lightheaded and felt generally crappy.

The nurse from the insurance company came over and we went through the whole thing again. She was nice, but it gets very tiring having to repeat it all the time.

My sister Terry is coming to Edmonton in December. We will have a family reunion, as her daughter, husband and two children will be here also. My brother Bernie and my sister Michelle and their families will also be here. It will be so nice to all be together. I hope God grants me the strength to enjoy it all.

Joanne and I made tourtières (meat pies) together. This is always a special time and an ongoing family Christmas time tradition. I could not undertake such a task alone yet and it's always more fun to bake together.

I went to see Dr. Tell (infection specialist) again. He was very interested in what Drs. Dare and Benhar had said and were doing. We talked for quite a long time. He said, "Annette, I still don't have answers for chronic fatigue syndrome patients at this time. Viral research is still ongoing." He looked at my rash again and asked if I had some on my wrists. He felt if the programs I was on helped, to keep them up and come back in February.

December 3, 1990

I'm not feeling too bad today, however my rash is bad on my hips, tummy and front of my thighs. It seems worse and I wonder if it's the toxins releasing as Dr. Dare said it might happen. Our skin is our largest organ and it does absorb and release things.

I've decided to go to a testing committee meeting on Thursday at work. I miss my work and I hope I can return in January. On the 5th I will be seeing Dr. Luck, a TMJ specialist.

December 7, 1990

On the 5th I went back to Dr. Benhar for another electronic diagnosis test. My allergies are better, however, my heart, circulation, kidneys, pancreas and cholesterol were not right according to him. He suggested walking for my circulation and felt my kidneys were trying to eliminate all the toxins and were having trouble handling it all. He gave me medication to clean my liver and kidneys and assured me things would improve.

I had lunch with Mom and then went to see Dr. Luck, the TMJ specialist. He seemed to think, from the beginning, that I likely had TMJ because of my overbite. An imprint was taken after a number of tests. If I went ahead it would cost approximately $300. We also discussed the clenching of my teeth and jaws at night. I had numerous questions for him. After so many doctors, I was skeptical of them all at first. I told him I would discuss this with Ken.

On the 6th I attended a testing committee meeting. It was so nice to see everyone, but I was drained by 11:30. I went to Drenda, massage therapist, and she said, "You look like you're in rough shape, let's go to work." She told me I had at least 10-15 lbs of accumulated fluids and suggested I drink parsley tea. I was not surprised by what she said. It seemed like I always felt "puffy" and had so much trouble loosing weight. I considered calling Dr. Tell and asking if I should try diuretics but decided I would try non-conventional treatments first.

December 20, 1990

Terry arrived from Montreal on the 11[th.] It's so nice to have her here. I had made appointments for her with Drs. Dare, Benhar and Tell. We found out that there was food we were both allergic to. It cost her $300 for everything so I do hope it helps her.

We managed to get our families together for a large meal and a very special time. I was so tired and the inflammation was bad. I knew I shouldn't get overtired but it had been worth it. Terry left on the 17th. It was hard to see my sisters and brother leave.

These days I'm bothered with a lot of pain in my thumbs and first fingers on both hands. It even hurts to hold a pencil. I've also have swelling and pain in my thighs. On days like this, I have to work hard at staying positive.

I called my department superintendent to talk about work. I have to face facts and realize I am not ready to return. He was kind and said he would talk to a teacher, who is replacing me, about continuing until spring break. I asked if I could go in once in a while to go through files or just visit to keep in touch. I was invited to come in any time. I'll have to see how things go month by month and think about part-time. It's very frustrating to know that I'm still so limited.

January 9, 1991

Christmas has come and gone once again. It was so special, but I'm feeling the effects of exertion and going off my diet.

Ken's colitis attacks seem to have lessened with the program Dr. Dare has him on. One of the things is high doses of vitamin C. I'm so glad to see him improve and in better spirits.

Some very interesting information has come my way regarding the location of my office at work. In approximately 1982/83, our department moved into a renovated wing in a junior high school. While I was there, many people were complaining of headaches, nausea, rashes and general ill health. We approached our department head about having the air quality checked, but he felt it was not necessary. This is also the time when I started to get ill. My office was located close to the furnace room and my desk was located next to the heating vents.

The week before Christmas 1990, people started to feel very ill, even slurring speech and fainting. They were also noticing a bad smell. The assistant superintendent called NorthWestern Utilities, who found the furnaces to have corroded air exchangers, and filters that had not been regularly changed, if ever (this information was obtained via my phone call to this company on January 8, 1991).

Also, I was told that the city gas department was called and informed that one furnace was especially unsafe and needed to be repaired immediately. I was stunned! What about the students and staff in the rest of the school? Had they been subjected to this pollution?

This was a breakthrough for us. My sister Terry, who had carbon monoxide poisoning, has similar symptoms to me. I called Drs. Tell and Dare to discuss these findings. If in fact this could have initiated my illness, I am furious. How could something like this ever happen, especially in a school with hundreds of children.

Gerda and I had lunch today and I'm thrilled I can do something like this. I'm looking forward to spending a quiet evening with Ken. Rachelle is going out with friends. Oh to be sixteen again!

February 3, 1991

On Tuesday I went to see Dr. Benhar (homeopath). He gave me drops for my lungs and kidneys. His diagnosis seems surprisingly accurate. My lungs were congested from a cold and my left kidney area was bothering me

Thank goodness for life's funny moments. That morning we brought our kitten Patches to be neutered. Before Christmas we had hurried to our veterinarian Dr. Herbers asking him to look at her. "She seems so sick," we said, "she keeps dragging herself on the ground and meows." He laughed and said, "She's not ill, but is definitely in heat." We all had a good laugh and thought for people who had so many animals, we were still learning.

This week I received a call from an assistant superintendent of another school system asking me if I would give a presentation to his councilors and special teachers. As it was to be at the end of February, I accepted. It would be a goal to look forward to and I would have plenty of time to review and prepare. Presenting on student evaluation has always been a pleasure and I missed it terribly. At the same time I hoped my health would permit me to do this.

One of the girls from work called and asked if I would talk to a gal named Donna, who had been ill for approximately 10 years with similar symptoms and facial pain. She and her husband were leaving for the same clinic that we had gone to. I advised her to go see Drs. Dare, Benhar and Luck and a good massage therapist before leaving. She did get an appointment with Dr. Dare today. We decided we would get together when she returned. She told me about another person who had been diagnosed with chronic fatigue syndrome. She apparently had been feeling considerably better since her amalgam (mercury) fillings had been replaced. This was interesting as Gerda went to see a dental specialist in Calgary, who had done research on the long-term effects of amalgam fillings. He told Gerda her mercury count was high and she is thinking of having her fillings replaced.

I keep going to Drenda, massage therapist, who helps me enormously. All this is costing us a bundle, but we have to keep trying to improve the quality of our lives. The vitamins, homeopathic medicines, consultations and therapeutic massage cost approximately $250-300 per month. I do hope we can manage without selling our acreage that we love.

I've written to our Health Minister, asking what her department is doing regarding preventive medicine and "non-conventional" medicine.

Again we are in an uncertain situation regarding Ken's work. Jobs are being cut and employees will be transferred to other locations. It looks like he may have a few options, but it may be very difficult to decide which way to turn, if in fact he is still employed. This is not helping our physical and emotional health. Regardless, we concluded that the only way to cope is to try being practical. We only have to open our eyes and realize there are many people worse off than us.

Last week I was at my office to pick up files and materials to review before the upcoming in-service I had agreed to do. Walking in was difficult and the tears were very near. How I missed being there! My love of children always left me wondering if their potential will be met. Will they be directed in a fashion that will enable them to achieve their potential? Will they feel good about themselves as they enter adulthood? These questions were always on my mind when working with evaluation tools.

Ken took a week off so that we could go to Calgary to see the same dental specialist that Gerda saw. We thought of it as a little "get away" that we desperately needed. We would stay with my sister and visit with them at the same time. It was only for a few days, but we were looking forward to it.

The morning of February 20 it started to snow. By the time we got to Red Deer (halfway) it was blizzard conditions. It was not a pleasant drive, at times so bad we had to follow truck taillights. Ken had a sinus infection that also affected his eyes. We managed to get to Calgary without an accident, very thankful to be there.

My consultation with the dentist was the next morning. Again I had to fill out a long questionnaire. He checked my mercury level. It was checked again after chewing gum for 10 minutes. The level was not as high as he thought, but it was most likely due to only three visible amalgam fillings. He was not able to tell if any of the bridgework and crowns had amalgam under them. He suggested that my symptoms indicated some form of toxic problem and that I should get the three fillings changed.

The test and consultation cost $75 (not collectable from our insurance company). Then we were on our way to look at some antique shops. Our stroll through the shops was short lived, as we both felt so ill. We decided to head back home to Edmonton, promising ourselves one day we would do this antique thing again.

That weekend I worked on the in-service to be given on February 26. I enjoyed putting it together, but I was very congested and my left side and back felt worse. On the day of the in-service I felt very faint and ill, but I was going anyway. I called the gal who was replacing me and she said she would drive us to St. Albert, as she wanted to attend the in-service. I was thankful but still had to get downtown. I prayed and asked my Dad in heaven to get me through the day, which I had so looked forward to.

We went for lunch and I decided to have two strong cups of coffee (remember I had not been drinking coffee). It would hopefully get the adrenaline going enough to carry me through the afternoon. I would have to deal with any consequences later. My heart was beating like crazy, but it worked. Although I was congested and my back was killing me, I made it through the day. The in-service was a success.

February 27, 1991

I called Dr. Benhar's office to see whether I should keep on with the homeopathic cleansers and decongestants. His nurse told me to stop taking everything and to drink a lot of water until I spoke with him. Ken stopped on the way home and bought me cranberry juice.

This morning I had an appointment with Dr. Mander (GP) for a gynecology examination. I mentioned my congestion and my sore side and back. He was surprised to find my lungs congested and said, "Yes, this time I can hear it." I reminded him that I had been congested for a number of years and had told doctors about it. He also suspected a bladder or kidney infection and found I had a yeast infection. I told him I had started Nystatin for yeast. He gave me a prescription for yeast medication. He said my bowels might be twisted again and ordered blood and urine tests. I was quite surprised that he seemed to treat me with respect and was genuinely caring and concerned this time.

For the last few days I have been putting heat on my back. I had a lot of very sharp pains and dull backaches. Today the pain has subsided a lot and I feel a little stronger. I'm singing and the cats are looking at me, as if to say, "What the heck has happened to her?" As I'm singing I think of how much I miss belonging to a choir. I hope I can one day sing with a choir again.

Dr. Benhar called last night and explained what had been happening was due to the homeopathic medications that he had put me on. He said, "Annette, your lungs are finally loosening up and you most likely passed kidney stones and impurities that account for the side and back pains. Keep drinking a lot of water, continue the drops and call me any time."

Rachelle will be leaving for Europe on a school trip March 22. She is excited and we are thrilled she is able to go. We recently found out Lorena and Robert are expecting again. What great news! I never thought that being a grandmother could be so heartwarming.

March 5, 1991

Dr. Mander called yesterday to say my cholesterol was still higher than normal, but not as high as before. Any improvement is good news for us. He called again tonight to tell me I had an estrogen imbalance and to use my 25 mg Estrogen patches every 3 days.

On the 7th I will be going to have my splint put in for TMJ.

March 11, 1991

On the 7th I went to Dr. Luck, the TMJ specialist. I was hooked up to a pulsator that was supposed to loosen my jaw muscles. It felt like my eyes were going to pop out of my head and I thought, "If this doesn't loosen my jaw muscles, nothing will!" I was then connected to a graphic-type machine that indicated how my jaw muscles functioned. My splint was then adjusted and after paying $150 (the other $150 to be paid later) I was on my way hoping for more miracles.

This is my fourth day and I must admit the ear noises don't seem quite as loud, especially during the day. The swooshing and pulsating is still there, especially at night. The pain in my left shoulder and neck doesn't seem as bad today.

I have started taking my temperature with a basal thermometer (under arm). Gerda was telling me that Dr. Kelm suggested this method to determine whether her thyroid was working properly. She lent me her thermometer for 3 weeks. On Saturday I didn't feel well and my temperature was higher than normal. Usually it stayed below normal. I don't understand how this temperature thing works, but it varies a lot and I'll talk to Dr. Benhar about it.

I've started drinking a Chinese tea that is supposed to "fill me with feelings of youth and beauty." If I could take the last 6 years away I might just have that feeling. "Think positive," I think, "Your second grandchild is coming and you want to enjoy your family." Tonight we are going to see Rachelle play piano in the Kiwanis Festival. Thank God for the blessings in life, they make the challenges tolerable.

March 25, 1991

The last few weeks have been up and down. The last few days have not been good. Financially, it's the pits! We seem to be getting behind with all we have to spend on vitamins, homeopathic medicine and therapeutic massage. I know I should cut back, but don't know where. These things help us and we need them. I hate this chronic fatigue syndrome/fibromyalgia, (the fibromyalgia diagnosis was recently added). I hate Ken's colitis and work situation. These situations are robbing us of our lives. We know it doesn't help to get discouraged. We remind ourselves that there has been improvement. At least, we know what were dealing with and there is a name attached to this illness. The conventional doctors don't seem convinced that it is what I have, but they don't have a name for me, do they?

I have decided to work 2 days a week. I pray things will be okay. I will meet soon with my employer to work out a schedule.

I have had my splint in for 2½ weeks. The noise is still there, although some of the pain has left, especially in my neck and shoulder. Rachelle is in Europe now, hopefully enjoying herself. We miss her; it seems too quiet here with her away.

April 3, 1991

On March 26 I went to see Dr. Kelm, Naturopath M.D., who now specializes in nutrition, vitamins and mineral therapy, Candida and hormonal therapy. I had discussed this previously with Dr. Dare and he agreed it would not hurt to see him.

I briefed him on what had been happening for the past 6 years. According to the temperature information that I shared with him, he readily suspected a low thyroid condition. He felt he could help me further by adjusting the supplements suggested by Dr. Dare. I asked about the evening primrose oil and he said, "Take as many as you can afford." His suggestions were Ester C, zinc, B6, calcium, magnesium, multi-vitamin/mineral, flax oil and ground flaxseeds. He decided not to give me a B12 shot at this time. He checked off a long list of blood tests to be done. It will be interesting to get these results back.

Joanne, my daughter, who is a Laboratory technologist specializing in hematology, was telling me that they hated to get Dr. Kelm's requests because they were so long. I told her that I appreciated the fact that he also worked with concrete results.

I had to complete another major questionnaire. He told me he would do a food analysis and in the meanwhile I should avoid whole wheat, coffee, tea, corn, peanuts, sweets and yeast and dairy products. I was to go on a 5-day rotation diet and keep taking my temperature.

Some of these foods I had already eliminated according to Dr. Benhar's (homeopath) suggestions. This would not be easy but I would do my best to stick by it.

I'd like to switch to the suggested vitamins and minerals, but I think I'll finish what I have first since money is not growing on trees these days. We discussed selling our acreage a few times, but I always end up wanting to stay, even if we have to scrounge. We would sell if all else failed.

I returned to Dr. Mander (GP) on the 27th, as I needed my Estrogen prescription renewed. He spoke to me briefly and decided I should go on 50 mg instead of 25 after I told him that I was still having symptoms.

I continue to see the massage therapist. She suggested cutting out more acidic foods, such as meats, pastas, any yeast products, honey and peanuts because my muscles and joints are so bad. I decided to try this and I was amazed after a few weeks how the pain had indeed lessened.

Yesterday I met with my department superintendent to discuss the hours of my work rehabilitation program. I will begin with working Monday, Tuesday and Thursday afternoons from 1 to 4 p.m. I am excited about going back to work and hope things work out well.

April 9, 1991

I seem to be improving on the adjusted vitamin and mineral program and everything else I'm doing. Today I was reading the Alive magazine and was interested in the body cleansing suggestions. Maybe I should give it a try. If I had toxins this might help. My brother Bernie had gone through an herbal cleansing and felt so well after. I imagine it is something most adults should do once or twice a year.

If toxins, accumulated mucous, undigested foods, etc. might contribute to cancer and serious diseases, why are cleanses not considered by the medical profession? Why can't Health Care consider preventative medicine? It only makes sense. Or, is it that the pharmaceutical companies run our Health Care system? After all, where would they be without sick people?

I started work last Thursday. I was a bit overwhelmed at first, mainly because my office seemed so different than when I had left it. I'm the type that needs things in order and have trouble working in an unorganized environment. I decided I would wait until summer to "tidy up."

I was amazed how clearly I could think. It was wonderful! I'll carry on for 3 afternoons a week for this month and if all goes well I'll then increase my time a little at a time. How nice it was to see my co-workers again.

I pray that God will continue to improve my health. How nice it would be to feel really healthy again. I'm so grateful for the help I've received and am convinced I'll keep improving.

I look at Ken and am so grateful for his love and support. I'll have to tell him again how I appreciate it. I've always known his and the children's love was there for me, but I imagine that being in such pain I may not have shown enough appreciation. I was so engulfed with one thing, survival!

How many people, I wonder, actually know anything about preventive medicine, good nutrition and non-conventional medicine. I wonder how we can be so ignorant about these things. Why is it not part of our educational system?

At times it is overwhelming. What to do and who to go to for help. There are so many non-conventional areas, like homeopathic remedies, reflexology, and holistic medicine in general. One wants to grab everything and anything that might help.

Today I'm at Joanne's. I've picked her up after she had her wisdom teeth extracted. It may sound funny that I'm mentioning this, but the fact that I can do this is so rewarding. She is not a complainer and I'm sure will soon feel fine. As I look at her sleep, I again thank God for the gift of my beautiful children. I'm so blessed to have them.

April 20, 1991

It seems like a lot has happened since I last wrote in my diary. The fact that I don't write in my diary as often is in itself good news that I'm improving.

On the 13th I went back to see Dr. Kelm. My food analysis report was not back yet, but we discussed my temperature readings. We discussed how I felt and I told him my leg muscle movements (vacillation) had lessened since I had increased my calcium and magnesium supplements.

163

He told me this was usually caused by the lack of magnesium. He started me on desiccated-liver thyroid pills. I was to take one every morning before breakfast until I saw him again on the 19th.

I thanked him for suggesting I work only 3 afternoons a week rather than 3 days. By the end of the afternoon I felt very tired. I shared with him that I had recently found out that the air quality was inadequate at Central Office, where our department was once again located. Carbon monoxide was coming back into the building. The vents are supposed to be fixed by the end of April. It boggles my mind how employers can be so thoughtless as to the condition of the working environment, thus endangering the health of their employees.

Terry called and it's always nice to share where we are with our respective health situations. Her doctors now are convinced that her problems were due to carbon monoxide poisoning. It is interesting that some of our symptoms are the same. We encourage each other and hope one day that we can be well again.

I went to Dr. Kelm to go through the food analysis. Taking into consideration it was based on 3 day's food intake, the findings were interesting. My salt intake was still high, even though I didn't salt anything. He explained it was the hidden salt in breads, sauces, etc.

I'm still going to Drenda, massage therapist. Her suggestion to eliminate some acidic foods has helped. To my understanding, if the acid is not excreted by the kidneys it can accumulate and form crystals in the joints and muscles.

It was suggested I drink much more water to help rid the body of these acidic crystals.

We are still waiting for our foal and can't believe how big Angel is. It should be born this week. Ken has gotten the birthing stall ready with the help of Robert and Dennis.

I've received an answer from our Health Minister. It was, as I expected, very brief. I was thanked for my suggestions regarding holistic and preventative medicine, but was informed that although we are free to pick and choose our medical help, alternative medicine was not yet recognized. Health Care would not cover any of these expenses. I was not surprised by the answer. This, to me, is not sensible or logical. How can government not be interested in saving millions of dollars by accepting and promoting preventative medicine? Other countries do this, why not ours?

May 10, 1991

The last few weeks have been rather incredible, to say the least. Along with everything else that was happening, our survival skills were tested even further. I share this with you, as an aside for the horse lovers who will understand.

On April 25 Angel had twin foals! Only one survived. That noon before leaving for work, I looked at her and noticed she was lying down in a strange position. I waited awhile and she got up and started grazing again, as usual. We had been watching her closely but could not see any real signs that she would soon foal.

That day Rachelle got home early and looked out her bedroom window and couldn't believe what she saw. There was a foal on the ground. In all her excitement, she didn't notice the other foal a little ways away, but it already had died. She quickly called the vet and covered the little foal, as it was a very cold and wet day. She tried to call Ken but he was in a meeting and my phone was busy. When we got home a short time later, we knew something had happened. Rachelle was very shaken and told us that Dr. Herbers had taken the colt to his clinic and shared everything that had happened. We hugged her and tried to reassure her that the vet would surely do everything he could to help the foal. It was a shame she had been alone and had done everything she could under the circumstances.

Reassured that the mare was okay, we all went to the clinic and met the most beautiful little foal. Big brown eyes looked at us and his coat was like velvet. He had been given medication and was now strong enough to suck milk from a bottle. At 11 p.m., we took him back home. Ken carried him, as he weighed only 33 pounds in comparison to a regular foal of about 50 pounds plus.

The next week was absolutely crazy! Ken and Rachelle milked the mare to feed him in the hopes that Angel would take him back when he was strong enough. We kept the foal in the laundry room of our new home. We bought rolls of plastic and used old blankets and straw.

For the first few days it was milk the mare, feed the foal and clean the laundry room. I could barely function and we were exhausted with this turn of events. Ken took time off, as there was no way I could cope.

On the third day we tried to re-introduce the foal to Angel. At first she seemed to accept him, then rejected him. He was so small and weak that it would be dangerous to leave him in the stall with her. Dr. Herbers suggested that we bottle-feed him. This would be difficult, as it meant months of bottle-feeding and Ken couldn't take too much time off.

Milking Angel was extremely difficult, so our vet got us some calf milk replacement. Poor little guy got severe colic and diarrhea. Back to the vet we went and he was given 2 shots and Pepto-Bismol. The vet bills were accumulating fast but we all agreed that we had to keep trying.

Once home we phoned a friend in Morinville who raised Morgan horses. We asked him if he knew anyone who might have a goat. He said, "It just happens that I have a mare that just lost a foal to the coyotes. Bring him here and we'll see if she'll accept him." If it works he said he'd lend us the mare for the summer. Our hopes were up.

At 11 p.m. we stopped at the vet's so he could give him another shot, which would help his colic until we got to Morinville, approximately 1½ hour away. We were both exhausted and I was so sore and tired that I could hardly see. Ken held him in the cab while I drove. At 1 a.m. we arrived and were so thankful that this couple were up and waiting for us. We prayed the mare would adopt him. We found that it was not to be. She knew it wasn't hers and wouldn't have anything to do with the colt. I walked out of the barn and cried. We were all disappointed and Roger invited us in for coffee and the foal lay on a blanket in the entrance. The coffee kept us awake for the ride back home. We got back about 4 a.m. and I had to go to work the next afternoon.

The next day Ken went to see if he could get cow's milk. The farmers said they couldn't spare any. He noticed a goat in a farmyard on the way home and thought, "What the heck, it's worth a try." We won't forget the lady's name, as she was so kind. Thelma gave Ken fresh goat milk to try. The goat milk worked! Although he still had diarrhea, he loved it and the rolling (indicating colic) stopped. Because Thelma needed the goat milk for her lambs, we found another couple near Tofield who raised goats. We were able to buy frozen goat milk. Unfortunately, they were only able to supply us with milk for a short period of time. In desperation, we advertised on a local radio station for help. The phone rang off the hook and people were very kind in offering all kinds of advice. A family, north of Westlock, offered to lend us their pet goat that had lost her kids.

We discussed this and opted to try the pet goat for a while. It would be much cheaper than buying frozen goat milk. After debating on a name for the colt, we called him Sonny. After all, we were his adopted parents.

Ken left to pick up the goat that day. He returned with a big bewildered Tiffany, the goat! She was not impressed with Tara, our Golden Retriever, and with one look at those horns she kept her distance. Milking Tiffany was another learning process and Ken decided he wasn't a farmer. She would walk up the little ramp and let Ken milk her or rather try to. She would look at him as if to say, "What in the world are you doing?" Then she would grab his hat. Eventually we got some milk, but it proved to be so much work and she wasn't giving much milk after a while.

A few months later Sonny was introduced to the outside world. He had his stall in the barn and eventually went out in the pasture. Sonny's legs were not strong and as he gained weight his front legs buckled and he would fall. We fashioned some leg braces and hoof pads for him, but it didn't help much.

His digestive system was still bothering him and we were beginning to think that we had been selfish to keep him alive. At that time Ken had been told he was being transferred to Calgary. Unfortunately, another move and one away from the children! Our daughter Joanne and her husband Dennis were kind enough to animal sit while we went house hunting. We were reluctant to leave them with this situation, but we had to go for a few days. Unfortunately, during this time Sonny passed away. It hurt us to know what Joanne and Dennis had gone through and wished we had been there instead When we look at pictures of him, we know we loved him dearly and did the right thing by trying to help him. A few years later, Angel gave birth to a healthy foal, which we named Bailey.

By the end of summer I knew that my chronic fatigue/ fibromyalgia was coming back with a vengeance.

September 19, 1991 (notes from diary)

For the last few weeks my feet have been swelling, especially the left one. This is frightening, as this is what had happened a few years ago at the start of my bad times. Now, at least, I know the name of this monster. Regardless, a set back is discouraging.

We decided to go see my brother Bernie and family in Fort McMurray. My left foot was really swollen, so much that I could barely get my shoe on. Massage therapy really helped, but at $35 a session I couldn't go every week. I went to see Dr. Dare and he felt it was part swelling and part fluid retention. And said it was a lupus-type of reaction. The lupus thing was coming up once again.

Before leaving I went to see Dr. Mander to see what he would say. He took a look and said, "I still think you have a collagen disease." Since when did he think this? I had never heard this before! He prescribed Endorphin, an anti-inflammatory. I started on the medication but the swelling continued and now my stomach was worse because of the medication. If I had the money, I would go back to Dr. Benhar (homeopath), but it's $150. Although we seem to be spending a fortune on supplements, I dream of the day that I'll feel well and go shopping and spend some of this money on clothing instead. If I do get something I need, I feel guilty buying it.

On the 28th I'll be 50 years old! Where has the time gone? It's hard to believe. There were days where I was sure I wouldn't see 50. Every day I thank God for my family, I love them dearly.

Drenda left for an extended period of time. I had to find another massage therapist. My new massage therapist suggested I should pursue a Chinese cleansing. Gerda told me about a yeast cleanse she is on. So many people are trying to help. I'll see what these are all about and should try anything that might help. Since this illness is chronic, I suppose it's a matter of trying things that might work.

September 25, 1991

I went to see Dr. Tell (infectious disease specialist) for a follow-up. I told him the anti-inflammatory pills didn't work. For a conventional doctor, he is very caring and personable. He listened and checked me over, measured my legs, and checked to see if an inside varicose vein or a blood clot could be causing the swelling. He said my blood pressure was a little high and felt it could be caused by fluid retention. He prescribed Dyazide, which is a mild diuretic. He said it shouldn't deplete my potassium. My cholesterol count was back to normal. The Dyazide seemed to help somewhat with the swelling for a time. But it came back again, regardless of the medications.

October 1991

As Ken had already started work in Calgary, I had to deal with the real estate agents and selling the house. We probably would have gotten more for it; however, we were nearing the end of time where Ken's employer would reimburse our moving expenses. The purchaser knew this and gave me a 2 a.m. deadline to consider the offer, and so it was sold.

In October we moved to Calgary. Also, Rachelle was leaving to model in Europe at this time. What an emotional time this was. The physical and emotional strain triggered all kinds of things in my body. It was so difficult leaving my children, mother, friends and work. The one thing that helped was that my younger sister lived in Calgary and I thought it would be an opportunity to get closer. Through it all, my older sister Terry was always there with encouraging words. Although far away, she never stopped helping me.

Finding new doctors, who would understand, was a worry. Everything that goes with relocation is always a challenge. Forever the optimist, I felt things would be okay.

For about 1½ years I stopped writing in my diary, thinking I was focusing too much on this illness and by doing this that I might improve. That was a mistake. I had many bad times and Ken, Rachelle and I faced many challenges that, with each other's support, we were able to get through somehow.

June 30, 1993

With this illness, I now realized a diary is usually necessary and often the only way to communicate one's feelings. Others can only listen for so long. I was faced with more illness and challenges. Ken's colitis was still giving him grief and I tried hard not to say too much. However, you'll see that with what I was experiencing it was hard to hide. The following is from my diary: "The last 6 weeks have been hell. I can't believe this is happening! It started with weakness and a black out, then diarrhea, and I felt really sweaty. I went to see Dr. Richard, my new naturopathic doctor in Calgary. He took blood work and said he thought it was a virus. Things did not improve, as I also got nauseated. I called him again but he was leaving for a 3-week holiday."

A few days later I experienced shortness of breath, faintness and my hand and feet got as cold as ice and I was shaking. Ken took me to the Clearview Hospital Emergency—a place I swore I wouldn't experience in Calgary. This surely was a nightmare... what were all these additional symptoms. I had a severe headache so a neurologist was called in. He took a few minutes with me and told me he didn't think it was neurological. He suggested that I should find a general practitioner because it was the best way to get medical assistance.

Back home I got worse and went to see Dr. Richard (naturopathic doctor). He still thinks it must be viral and things have got to improve shortly. Back home I do my relaxation and visualization and pray. I think God is too busy to reach down to me.

Things get even worse! I can't eat and I'm constantly nauseated. The doctor, suggested by the emergency doctor, is not seeing new patients so I saw another young doctor who really was at a loss.

By the third week I'm having more attacks and they were increasingly severe. One night it was so bad that we went back to emergency. The lady doctor is sympathetic and has x-rays and ultrasound done and sends us home.

Ken called the hospital administrator to ask what we should do. As well, he asked for the name of a highly recommended doctor. We were given the name of Dr. Fisher. I made an appointment for Monday, July 12. Things are not improving so I called Dr. Fisher's Office and they were able to see me a couple days earlier. He readily suspects a blockage in the digestive system and books me for a barium test.

That night I again experience a terrifying attack. My stomach was distended, I felt nauseated and like I was going to faint. It woke me up out of a deep sleep. Back to emergency we went!

"How could you get stuck with someone like me?" I yell at Ken. The same lady doctor looks after me and I'm booked into the hospital under Dr. Fisher.

July 13, 1993

I don't know if I should be glad, they might help. I look around and I want to run away, far away, to a place where there's no pain and doctors! This is a reoccurring deja vu. It is different symptoms, in addition to some of the fibromyalgia symptoms.

As I'm given an upper barium test, the radiologist tells me he can see a loop in my bowel. I think, "Finally they have found what is making me so ill." A gastro resident takes my history and the next morning Dr. Loges (G.I. specialist) comes to see me. He thinks that a loop in my upper bowel shouldn't cause all my symptoms and they decide on another ultrasound and book me for an endoscopy. I also have an ECG.

I pray for help because I think I'm going to "loose it." I'm so scared. I have to put all this in God's hands. I try to do my relaxation and deep breathing to fall asleep. I'm on an I.V. and clear fluids. The attacks still come, but not as severe. I'm given oxygen for a few nights.

The results from the endoscopy come back normal. No growth or ulcers, but I'm told they weren't able to get to the duodenum where the problem is suspected.

Dr. Loges (G.I. specialist) came in with some interns and said, "You see my nose is bigger than yours (he had that right), well my intestines are different than yours. Just because there are a few abnormalities it doesn't mean that's what causing you to be so ill."

"Oh no," I thought, "I don't believe this. Here is another person that shouldn't be a doctor." Because he could not come to a conclusion or didn't want to be bothered to continue, he felt better making me feel and look a "fool." This was becoming another nightmare! It would not take much to give up at this point. I cry myself to sleep and pray a miracle can happen.

After 10 days, the barium still hasn't passed and is lodged at the entrance of my large bowel. A young nurse is sent in—this is to be her first enema! To make a long story short, she doesn't take the cap off the tube before inserting it into me. I knew something was wrong because she kept coming back and "fiddling around." The head nurse comes in and explains, all apologetic. She tries also and can't get the cap out. By this time, I'm not impressed and getting embarrassed. I tell her, "Give me a glove and I'll get the darn thing out," and I did. As I sat on the toilet, I laughed and cried. Where was my sense of humor? At another time this would be funny. Somehow it wasn't.

Poor Dr. Fisher (GP) was so distraught about everything and was not impressed with the old G.I.'s comment. He booked me for a test where they were to put a tube down my stomach to look at the inside. But three x-rays later and many enemas, the barium still hadn't moved out! I'm given some stuff called "Go Lightly"—not an appropriate name. I'm to take a gallon of this stuff? How, I ask, when I can't even swallow a cup of fluid? I take three large glasses and feel very ill and burp a salty solution all the next day. The barium moves enough that the test will be done on the 26th. I sleep and dream that I'm a child and I'm running away and frightened.

The test was terrible! After three tries the tube is finally put down my nose to my stomach and to my small intestine. As the tube was being pushed through, it stopped near the duodenum and the female radiologist said, "The tube can't be put through there without pushing it hard." They then discussed the severe narrowing. Barium was put in and another bunch of pictures taken. I'm sure by now that I'm positively radioactive. They comment on the bowels being out of place, loops and scarring and narrowing. I'm glad this is nearly over, maybe now someone will help me.

I'm very bloated and nauseated since the test. Dr. Fisher (GP) comes in and said he had talked to the radiologist and the conclusion was it wasn't severe enough for an operation.

"What was I to do?" I asked him. "I need help." I was released from the Clearview Hospital still very ill and on clear fluids. I was told to see Dr. Fisher on Thursday (2 days away). I came home frightened and Ken was furious. I couldn't blame him. I called Dr. Richard (naturopathic doctor), as he was now back and made an appointment with him also on Thursday.

Dr. Fisher saw me and couldn't give me any explanation, although he still suspected I somehow couldn't process my food. He told me to add some cream soups and full fluids, if I could, and come back in a week.

Dr. Richard was astonished how I looked. I had weight loss, was white as a sheet and so weak. I told him the story and he said it sounds like your thyroid is hardly functioning and he felt my body was going into some sort of shock. He couldn't believe the barium had stayed in me so long. I was told to have an enema as soon as I got home. We discussed the thyroid and I explained they said at the hospital that it was within the normal range. He asked me to start on two natural thyroid pills a day.

He asked me to call and tell him how they made me feel. I called the next day and said I was not well— bloated, shaky and feeling faint. I am alone today and it's frightening. I can't expect everyone to drop what he or she is doing, just for me. I'm happy Rachelle is gone to Wabamum Lake; she needs the distraction, as she's looking tired.

This afternoon I tried to eat three bites of tuna and rice. I'm so weak that I feel I have to try eating. It didn't make me feel better. I feel worse! "Think positive, think positive," I cry out. I can't give up. I know eventually that I'll get help. Also, I'm dealing with symptoms of chronic fatigue/fibromyalgia. I think I've had enough and wonder why I have been chosen to experience yet another nightmare so soon. I cry and cry... there are no more tears left.

July 31, 1993

Robert, Lorena and grandchildren came to visit yesterday. It is so special to see them all. We made supper and I ate a bit of green beans, potato and some butter lettuce from the garden. It tasted so good, but I felt like I had eaten a huge meal and was bloated and burping my little supper at 2 a.m. Despite of it, I had a pretty good sleep that I desperately needed.

In the morning I had a bit of toast and oatmeal. Now an hour later, I feel weak and bloated. It's like it won't go through my system. I get so frustrated and wonder why, when it comes to me, nothing is medically black and white.

I look in the mirror and I look like a ghost, I'm so white. I call Dr. Richard and ask if it's the thyroid and how long it will take to work. He said, "By Christmas we'll have you feeling like new." Christmas! That's 5 months away. Nothing, but nothing, is as bad as ill health.

August 4, 1993

Things are always the same. I went to my sister Michelle's for Mom's birthday. Mom had ordered Chinese food that looked so good. I had a bit of lemon chicken and rice and suffered all night. It feels like I have a ball in my stomach most of the time.

August 6, 1993

I went to see Dr. Fisher (GP) for a follow-up. He didn't say much, except that I might be "too aware of my body." Here we go again, the one doctor I thought might eventually help with this digestive problem. Asked if he felt it might be part of chronic fatigue, he said, "All this chronic fatigue/fibromyalgia stuff is fairly new and the diagnosis is questionable. I couldn't tell you if it is."

On Saturday I went outside to weed in the garden. I have to keep going. I find if I sit every ½ hour or so I can keep going. My muscles are sore. I'm shaky and tired and my stomach is still foreign, but I'm so proud to have accomplished a little weeding.

Ed and Gerda, our friends, stopped on their way home from Lake Louise. She looks great! It's so nice for them that she's feeling better. I'll try and find a chiropractor that does the Nucca method, which straightens the spine by adjustment of the axle vertebrae. There has got to be more answers out there.

On Sunday I was able to go to church. I asked God why this is happening and could he help us deal with what comes our way. Again, I plead for answers and help.

In the afternoon we went for a drive to Kananaskis Country with Mom, my sister Michelle and her husband Ron. It is a beautiful and peaceful area in the mountains. Mom is not feeling well and it's always special to spend time with her, when I'm able to.

September 5, 1993

Most of August was spent going to Dr. Richard. He started me on Zantac for my stomach and low dosage of Ativan to help me sleep. I took a ½ Ativan only if I could not get to sleep or woke up with problems.

On Monday, the 6th Rachelle asked if I would like to go with her to the University so she could register. I really wanted to do things that were "normal." According to some doctors I should be "okay."

It wasn't a good idea! I was standing in line with her, talking and thinking how nice it would be to take a few courses when I suddenly felt weak. Excusing myself, I went to sit on the stairs. I asked a lady in a nearby office if she could get me some juice. I knew I was borderline hypoglycemic, but had eaten before leaving. Apologizing, I asked Rachelle if we could go home when she was finished. I just couldn't tour the University as planned.

On Tuesday I tried to get up, but felt like fainting. I tried a few times, then called Michelle and asked if Ron would mind driving Mom over. I was so happy to have her with me for the day.

Winter 1993/94

That winter was a matter of going to Drs. Fisher and Richard and trying to cope with chronic fatigue syndrome and major digestive problems. Dr. Richard still suspected it had to be associated with a systemic disorder and gave me some intravenous treatments of vitamins and other supplements. My strength improved a bit, but I still struggled with major digestive problems. An enlarged blood vessel was found in the liver during an ultrasound. This, they felt, was insignificant and would not cause my symptoms.

Playacting became a part of my life. I challenged myself to pretend things were "okay" when family and friends were over. It was harder with Ken because he would see the frustration and would be there at night when I woke up so ill. In addition, we had to cope with other stresses that life would bring. I don't know how we could have made it without the support of good friends, family, and our children and grandchildren.

May 20, 1994

Mom has moved to Calgary, as she is not well. She has congestive heart failure and it's so hard to see her so ill, when she loves life so much. She has taken a small apartment, but I don't think she'll be there long. I worry about her coping on her own. We phone each other often and I help her out as much as possible.

Today I write in my diary again because I can't discuss a lot of my discomfort and pain, even with Ken. He's truly fed up, I can tell. I have intermittent constipation and diarrhea, severe pain in my upper left side. I'm burping, or rather trying to, because I'm so bloated. Dr. Richard felt we should get another opinion from Dr. Stein (Gastro). I had a long wait for his appointment and I ended up seeing him in emergency. He gave me a prescription but I don't see any change. In fact, I feel more bloated on it. I'll keep going and won't give up. Some day I'll feel better and enjoy life like I so want to. Through all of this, it is important to count one's blessings, such as family, children, grandchildren, good friends and faith. I was going to add sense of humor, but it gets harder and harder to add humor to this.

September 1994

I'm trying intravenous hydrogen peroxide treatments suggested by Dr. Richard. It can kill infections and viruses. For a few days after the treatments, I felt remarkably well in comparison to before. I then came down with a bad flu that knocked me back down again.

When the flu subsided Ken and I thought a few days away somewhere might help me, but we have so many medical expenses that I don't think it will happen. I should get more chelation treatments.

As I suspected and kept telling dentists, an infection was discovered in the tooth that I recently had a root canal done. It will have to be redone and the cost will be $1,000 over our insurance. I feel so discouraged that I can't help provide and am unable to collect any disability benefits, as chronic fatigue or fibromyalgia is not yet recognized as a disability. I call it the modern day disorder that is now increasing in large numbers.

December 1994

Somehow we got through the special season of Christmas. The children were unable to come to Calgary so we went to Edmonton. The holiday season was special but also it was sad because we knew Mom would not be with us next year at this time. She was now on oxygen and very ill. My chronic fatigue was like a roller coaster and my digestive problems still horrible. Doctor appointments continued but things basically stayed the same. Mom had seen a very good Internist by the name of Dr. Mendally. I thought that it might be beneficial to make an appointment with him, especially about my serious digestive problems. In order to do this, I had to again go though my general practitioner or Dr. Richard.

May 1995

I've been dealing with sharp pain in my lower abdomen and groin. It starts with a very sharp pain in the right groin and it leaves numbness in the groin and towards my hip. Dr. Fisher (GP) thought it might be a torn adhesion. He told me if it got worse to return. It did and a CAT scan was done of the abdomen and pelvis area. He explained that the films were not clear because of all the adhesions from previous surgeries (e.g., appendicitis, hysterectomy and ovarian cyst). He again thought it to be a torn adhesion and told me to place a book on the sore spot and wrap myself with a tensor bandage.

To this day it still bothers me. The numbness is better but I get pain at this site—approximately where the barium (entrance of the large bowel) stayed lodged for so long!

June 1995

That month we lost our Mom. It was so hard saying goodbye, even if we knew she was better off in God's arms and with her dear husband Philippe. Rachelle said "Now we now have double the power from heaven because both Grandpa and Grandma are there." Our Rachelle is wise beyond her years.

The rest of the summer was like a daze. I never realized how much I would miss my parents now that they were both gone. I found myself thinking, "I have to phone Mom and tell her this or ask her that." I felt her presence near me and knew my parents still love and watch over us.

I was so thankful for good friends and neighbors like Nancy, Deanne, Marjo and Elaine and John. I knew they were there and would always help us. We learned it isn't the quantity of friends, but rather the quality that counts. I feel so blessed for the special friends that have cared for me enough to share their time with me. It's a rare gift to have a special friendship.

October 19, 1995

Dear Diary, please let me share with you again. I'm so torn; I want to write but feel at times if I do, I focus too much on illness.

All last night I was sick. I was going to call Rachelle because Ken was gone to Medicine Hat. He has been traveling a lot since our move to Calgary. I think it's most likely good for him to get away. I decide to let Rachelle sleep, as she needs her rest and, like everyone around, must be tired of her sick mom. I'm having so much trouble digesting. I ate a small supper at 5 p.m. and I'm still burping it at 3 a.m.

Friday, October 20, 1995

By September I'm experiencing severe attacks, especially at night. My abdomen hurts on the left and around my rib cage and then bloats. I have to burp, but I can't. Then my body starts to shake and I get very weak. The pulsating noises in my head seem worse. God, I'm thinking at times I want to join my parents with everlasting peace and no more pain and discomfort. I scold myself for thinking of such a thing, but it's been on my mind more and more lately.

I called Nancy, my friend and also a nurse, to pick me up and bring me to the hospital. Meanwhile Marjo, friend and neighbor, stayed with me until Nancy came. I was so weak and shaky that I could hardly get to the phone to call them.

Nancy picks me up and stays with me at emergency. Dr. Mendally (Mom's Internist), who I had finally made an appointment to see at his office, was at the hospital. He suspected an obstruction and wondered about blood flow to the abdomen. He calls Dr. Benoski (Gastro Surgeon), who also wants to check for a possible abdominal tumor because of my symptoms. He assures me, "We'll get to the bottom of this."

Nancy prays with me that God will enlighten these doctors and help me. I look at her and thank her for being my friend.

Dr. Benoski wonders whether I should go home and see him next week. Nancy intervenes and tells him how ill I am and that it's too frightening to be home and that I can't continue this way. He agrees and admits me to the Layco Hospital.

Dr. Benoski doesn't want to repeat the CAT scans, if he can view the ones at the Clearview Hospital. He tells me a number of tests will be done to eliminate things before he decides to operate. At this point I just want help.

Rachelle came at 5 p.m. It is hard to put up a strong front for here. In the evening she returns with some things I need. I lie there at night and suddenly realize that I must be living a continuous medical nightmare. Am I really hospitalized again? Will someone really help me this time?

I try positive visualization and see Rachelle, Ken and I riding along a beautiful trail with the sun setting. I can smell the fresh air and see fields and trees. I fall asleep but wake in the night and cry.

I would love to see the children from Edmonton but I don't want them to know I'm in the hospital again. I pray that the findings this time will be of a helpful nature.

Friday, Ken came back from Medicine Hat at 3 p.m. and stayed until 5 p.m. As discouraged as he looked, it was so nice to have him beside me.

Dr. Benoski said nothing much would happen on the weekend. He asked me to try liquids. At 8 p.m. I had some apple juice and a bit of water. My side started to hurt and bloat a short time later. I had a very bad night. I could not lie down and tried to sleep in the chair. At 1 a.m. I tried a bit of grape juice. The pulsating in my head and body was very bad. At 4 a.m. the nurse brought me some Ginger

Ale. I burped a bit but was more bloated afterwards and I sat in a chair until sunlight came through the window.

Saturday, October 21, 1995

My urine is being collected for 24 hours. Two hours before completion it is accidentally thrown out, so I have to start over. I'm so tired from the attacks and bad night. My left side is continually bloated and hurts. I tried having a bit of liquid porridge and some coffee at 8 a.m. At noon, when my broth soup arrives, I'm still burping my porridge.

I called Rachelle and told them not to bother coming to the hospital. I would rather see them doing other things than sitting here. In the morning Rachelle came and helped me take a shower. I can't believe how weak I am! Ken came in the afternoon and we played cards. What a difference it made to have them with me.

That night I thought of how long that we had been struggling with my illness, over 10 years with one thing or another. I think of how ill I've been during my life and wonder why I have been so blessed. Apparently, life and challenges makes one stronger. It would be nice to have a break now and again. "Now I'm feeling sorry for myself," I think. There are many people much worse off than I am. I say my rosary and pray also for others that are lonely and sick and ask God to help us.

Sunday, October 22, 1995

Last night was not much different than other nights. All night I kept sitting up to try burping my salty broth I had for supper the night before. The nurse told me to mention this to the doctor when he came in.

The "generic" weekend residents came by. From the look of the "leader of the pack," he's not too worried and is not impressed by what I say. I tell him that I'm still bloated from the broth and I'm still burping it. He shakes his head and grins at the other two guys with him. He says, "I would not know what causes it. Nothing much happens here on weekends." "You're telling me," I think. I'm informed that no one has looked at the x-rays from the Clearview Hospital yet and I'm told to "hang in there," my doctor should be in tomorrow.

The nurse comes in shortly after and says he's ordered Magnesium Citrate to "clean me out." I told her of my last experience with this stuff. I ask if they could do an enema instead, as I really hadn't eaten anything since last Wednesday. She tells me she's sorry but that's what the young doctor ordered.

I'm in tears when she leaves and I decide to fight this time. As a patient, I try to treat the staff with respect. Seldom have I gotten angry like I was now. Before I had a chance to call her, Dr. Benoski's assistant came in and I explained to him the problem that I had the last time I took Magnesium Citrate. He said, "It's not necessary, we'll use something else for the test." Today my left side hurts constantly and it goes all the way to the back. When I got up this morning, it felt like I had a ball in my stomach and I had shooting pain from the abdomen up each side of my throat and into my ears. I knew I had to burp to get relief so I asked the nurse for some Ginger Ale. The pain subsided after about 5 minutes. I had never had anything like this before, but by now wasn't surprised at anything. I try to do positive imagery but find I can't concentrate. I just want this over. I want to feel good! I'm so tired of all this, I think I'm going to go insane. "Stop!" I tell myself. Think of something good, anything. I see my children and think back when they were little and how proud I am of all of all their accomplishments. How lucky I am to have them. Then there's Ken who keeps supporting me, although I'm sure at times he'd love to go on a one-way trip. If we move to Lethbridge, I will dearly miss our amazing friends and neighbors we have in Calgary. The stress of moving again will not improve my health, but one does what one has to do.

So far, I had not wanted Ken to tell Joanne and Robert I was hospitalized again. I suppose after being here a week, we should tell them. There is absolutely no improvement and I'd love to see them. Sometimes I wonder how long a body can go like this. I come to the conclusion that mine can take a lot before giving up.

Monday, October 23, 1995

Last night I was given an oral laxative medication. As much as I have been saying I can't take these, I am told I have to take them. Once again, I got very bloated and very ill. By 11 a.m. it hasn't improved.

(Notes from diary)

"God I'm so sick, please give me the strength to deal with what comes my way." I want to give up but I know I can't. What are they missing? How can the medical profession do this to anyone? If this is happening to me—what is happening to others? I have to write my story to help others and make the public aware of what can happen. "God I can't handle this, please help me!" I'll have to ask for some form of counseling soon.

It's 11:45 a.m. and I'm still waiting to be taken for that darn barium enema. While I wait, I look out the window at the people walking and pretend I'm amongst them and I'm rushing to meet a friend for a lovely lunch. I can taste the food and imagine I'm eating eggs benedict and chatting with Marjo, Nancy or Elaine over lunch. Maybe today it's with Deanne, or maybe, Gerda or Linda who have come to Calgary. We've been shopping and are now having lunch.

My thoughts are suddenly interrupted when someone comes in to take me to my test. Before they start I'm given an x-ray and told they can't do it because I still have barium in my intestines from last Wednesday. I can't believe it! I'm in tears as they wheel me out.

Dr. Benoski (Gastro Surgeon) and his team of residents come in and he says they had gotten the x-rays from the Clearview Hospital and would look at them. He tells me I should have another prep to try to get rid of the lodged barium. I just look at him and can't say anything. He continued to tell me he didn't think it was a thyroid problem and wanted to eliminate the adrenal tumor possibility. "Unfortunately," he then added, "you then will have been checked by two major hospitals. We can open you up, but I'm not sure that we'll find anything, except adhesions." Oh God! I'm sure they think I'm nuts again. It's apparent by the comments and the way they look at each other.

I'm also beginning to think that I'm nuts. Also, that someone is wishing me ill. What can it be? I don't want an exploratory operation.

October 24, 1995

Now, I'm only on I.V. and my night seemed a little better. I'm not as bloated and sore. Rachelle was here in the morning and we had a good talk. Dr. Benoski came in and said the CAT scan from the Clearview Hospital didn't show anything and they didn't have the results of the urine test yet. He felt he should operate to see what was going on inside. When he comes in without the residents he seemed much more professional and caring.

Now it's back to the x-ray department. As I wait in the same room I waited with Mom, I feel her presence and wish she could be here to hold my hand. I'm told they still can't take it, as the barium is still there. They can't understand with all the stuff and enemas that I've been given, that somehow it hasn't moved. This is no longer funny and this time no one jokes about it. It is lodged in my ileum secum valve, which is between the small and large bowel.

In the afternoon Deanne and Marjo are in for a visit. Nancy called and we had a good talk. I thank God for them. It's evening and I'm given more enemas. The days are endless, without any food breaks to change the monotony. I'm feeling so weak and having to stay in bed a lot makes the days even longer. Thank God for books, family and friends.

Ken comes in later and looks so tired. He's so busy at work and has to cope with this, as well as his colitis. During the night I wake up to find the I.V. fluid running into the tissues and my arm was swollen and painful. Unfortunately another I.V. needle had to be inserted.

October 25, 1995

This morning they gave me another enema and I feel so weak. Down to x-ray again I went. It still showed a little barium but they decided to go ahead and put more barium in me for the test!! To this day I still have problems with this valve. As I lay there cold and weak, I wondered again what I had done to deserve this and the tears fell.

Later that morning Dr. Benoski told me he was glad nothing was found in the lower bowel. Now it would be harder to find out what was wrong. He asked me to try a little solid food again to see what would happen.

Ken came after work. I look at him and love him for the support and caring he gives me. He made me a toast and brought me half a pear. I ate it at 7:30 and by 8:30 I was ill. All the symptoms were back. I was bloated and had so much pain. My night was very bad!

Thursday, October 26, 1995

It's been a week since I was admitted. I'm trying to keep my sanity, but I'm not doing well. More and more when the residents came in, it seemed like my illness was a big joke. After eating that toast I was so ill and depressed that a nurse came and sat with me for a while. Yes, there is some compassionate and understanding medical personnel around. I mentioned that I sometimes wondered if it could be neuro-gastro. She said her father-in-law had that and felt it was worth mentioning to the doctor. When the weekend "generic" doctors came in, I told them what a bad night I had after eating that toast. The head resident grinned and said, "Well, all your tests seem okay so far. We'll probably discharge you today and make an appointment with Dr. Mendally (Internist) for you." I mentioned the neuro-gastro thing and they looked at each other and grinned. I look at them and can't believe these guys are to be doctors taking care of human beings when they lack respect, compassion and have no communication skills.

I told them I wanted to see Dr. Mendally before being discharged. I was told that would be just about impossible, as he was "hard to get a hold of." The head resident looked annoyed and they left. I heard them laughing when they got to the hallway. At that moment I wanted one of them to experience my pain, discomfort and frustration for a day.

I called Ken and he agreed I should see Drs. Mendally and Benoski first. How could I cope when I couldn't eat? I just couldn't justify having major surgery without knowing what it was for. I called the head nurse and informed her I could not leave without seeing Dr. Mendally first. I told her of the resident's attitudes and she said she would talk to Dr. Benoski about them.

Dr. Benoski came in and we discussed what had happened. I also told him that Ken and I weren't impressed that a resident could make such major decisions. He then told me he felt we should operate and that he would get Dr. Heart's (another surgeon) opinion. He talked about all the tests that had been done at the two major hospitals. "Here we go again," I thought. He added, "I'm not one for saying let's look at the psychological aspect, but that might be an option." I told him I had seen two psychologists and kept seeing one, once in a while, to help me cope with my medical situation. The psychologist had assured me that the only thing wrong was the stress from all this medical B_ _ _ S_ _ _ and that I was perfectly sane.

Dr. Benoski then said, "Dr. Mendally suggested another test. It involves you eating a radioactive egg sandwich and then following it through for 3 hours." I remembered Dr. Mendally mentioning this rather unusual test the first time I went to see him. I had forgotten about it and now asked why it hadn't been done before.

In the afternoon I had the test. It was very difficult because after an hour I started to bloat and felt very sick. And there it was, still sitting in my stomach after 3 hours. The x-ray technician was surprised but I wasn't. I had been telling doctors this for a long time.

Ken and Rachelle were here in the evening. When I see them I miss home so much. Rachelle was making us laugh. She blew up a rubber glove and wrote on it: "Enter at your own risk. Enema Zone!"

It's now 8:30 p.m. and I'm still bloated from the egg sandwich that I ate at noon. I got to sleep listening to tapes and saying my prayers. I pray for my family and friends and that God grant me some answers and help soon.

Friday, October 27, 1995

Dr. Benoski (gastro surgeon) suggested he operate. He had consulted with Dr. Heart, who had looked at the latest test results and felt there was a blockage of some sort and that surgery was the only route to try to help me. Dr. Heart came in and explained this to me. Now here was a surgeon who had chosen the right path in life. He was kind, soft spoken and obviously knew what he was talking about. I wished that he had been more involved in my case.

193

Surgery is always a big decision and I prayed I would make the right decision. I couldn't stay the way I was and the next step was to try something that might help me. It was scheduled for the next day, which was Saturday. That they would operate on a Saturday surprised us, but I was glad I didn't have to wait until Monday.

October 28, 1995

I was frightened as I waited in the hallway alone to go into surgery. The anesthetist came to talk to me and told me what he would do. By the time I was wheeled in, I was shaking, most likely from fright rather than cold. I asked God to be with me and help the surgeon find what was making me so ill and hopefully fix it.

As I was being put to sleep, the nurse explained that she had to press hard on my throat. I remember it being very uncomfortable, and the last thing was counting and the horrible taste and smell of the anesthesia and the operating room.

When I woke up, I was in my bed and Ken was there. I don't remember much of the first day, except I had all kinds of tubes, a catheter and special stockings for blood circulation. The tube in my nose was hurting my throat a lot and I hoped I wouldn't have to keep it long. Rachelle came to see me and Ken stayed that night and the next.

October 30, 1995

On the 29th, the day after surgery, the nurses had me sit up and stand by the bed. It felt like I was tearing open. I wasn't alarmed as I had surgery before and I knew how it would feel when I first tried to get up. They took the stockings off and I was able to move my legs and that felt good. Then the catheter was taken out. As far as I was concerned, the more tubes that went, the better off I would be. The tube was really hurting my throat so I tried to sleep with the bed up most of the night. Again for the third night, Ken stayed with me and slept in the chair.

October 31, 1995

Halloween and I won't be there to carve the pumpkin! For the past 36 years the kids and I have carved a pumpkin together. Rachelle and her friend Isabelle carved a huge one that Ken had bought. I told Ken to stay home that night and get some decent sleep.

November 1, 1995

The doctor decides to take the tube out as fluids are going through. God, I'm so happy, as it is such a relief not to have it! I'm told to start drinking liquids. He drew a picture of what he had done—a pyloroplasty (a procedure that tilts the pylorus at a different angle to let the food out of the stomach). After completing this procedure, they checked my intestines and discovered ulcer scarring by the duodenum that had resulted in a severe narrowing. This was probably the main reason that my food wouldn't go down and the pyloroplasty surgery may not have been necessary. They quickly scraped the scarred area and also untwisted my intestines in three places. No wonder I would bloat. He explained they didn't have much time to do the scraping of the scarred area, as I had been under for 2 hours already and hoped it would "do the trick."

November 2, 1995

The residents came in. I really hate it when they come into my room. They don't seem to take anything seriously and tell me I'm most likely going home the next day. I can't believe I'm hearing this after major surgery and I'm on water, juices and I.V. I told the residents I was anxious to get home but felt it was too early. I had just started on clear fluids and felt I should know if I could eat. I didn't want to land up back here. They kept grinning and saying how "good" I looked. Yes, I was sure I looked great after what I had been through.

When they left I just shook my head and thought, "Is this a result of our current Health Care cuts? Cut them up, sew them up and ship them home to deal with whatever happens."

My son Robert was here to see me from Edmonton. What a nice surprise! He brought pictures of Daniel and Marc and we had a nice visit. I assured him I'd be fine now that the blockages had been fixed.

Friday, November 3, 1995

This morning Dr. Benoski and his "followers" came in laughing. I was combing my hair in the bathroom. He said, "Well, I want you to feel comfortable about going home today." As he says this, he is about to burst out laughing and the residents are laughing so much that one has to leave the room. I ask them to please share the joke so I could also have a laugh. They just look at one another and grin. "What a bunch of unprofessional medical personnel!"

I answer that if the big joke is that I don't feel ready to leave until my body can cope with full fluids, then I don't find anything amusing in that at all. I tell them if they feel I should be discharged, then I wanted the I.V. out now and I would leave after having full fluids at supper.

They left. As the tears fell, I swore I'd never be back! What difference would a day make? I should stay at least a week or long enough to make sure I could eat. Was that not the concern for so very long?

I was told by the dietitian to have cream soups, cream of wheat and Ensure (a liquid meal substitute). I left after eating my first bowl of cream soup and jello. I felt full, like I'd eaten a huge meal.

I was so happy to be home again. I looked around and cried. I went to bed feeling very weak and bloated.

Saturday, November 4, 1995 (notes from diary)

It is now a week today since I had my surgery. Joanne and Dennis are coming today and I'm looking forward to seeing them. I'm trying to drink Ensure and take full fluids, but I'm just feeling more and more bloated. My stomach is visibly distended. I'm not able to visit much with the kids, as I feel so weak that I'm in bed most of the time.

Sunday, November 5, 1995

Took a bit of cream of wheat for breakfast but it didn't seem to want to go down. At lunch I tried to drink some Ensure but could only take a sip or two. Joanne and Dennis left after supper and it was so hard to see them leave. I couldn't drink anything at all and eventually vomited everything I tried to put down.

Monday, November 6, 1995

In the morning I threw up again. Ken and I headed for the Layco Hospital Emergency at about 11 a.m. I was so weak I couldn't walk. Dr. Benoski was called and he sent me home with a prescription for motility pills. They didn't do anything! I kept vomiting even if I didn't eat; my stomach juices now wouldn't even go through. By 6 p.m. I was still vomiting and was seeing double. I was so dehydrated. I felt like I was dying! Crying, I looked at Ken and told him that I loved him and to love the children and grandchildren if I died. We went back to emergency and I was admitted to a different surgery floor—very, very ill.

Tuesday, November 7, 1995

Ken and I looked at each other and cried. I would bloat and vomit. Why did this have to happen? We knew I had been discharged too quickly. I should have been on clear fluids longer and monitored before adding full fluids.

Wednesday, November 8, 1995

We were now told that it was a total blockage and it could be post-surgical inflammation or "something of that nature." I was so weak from vomiting, and could hardly function. I was then put on I.V.

Thursday, November 9, 1995

I was taken down for a barium swallow x-ray but could not even take a few swallows because I was so bloated. I now carried a bowl with me at all times. The x-ray showed I had a blockage by the duodenum just before the small intestine, the area that they had scraped some of the ulcer scarring away. My stomach was now stretched to twice the size.

This afternoon I had an endoscopy to see if they could determine the cause. I came back from the test coughing and my hair and gown covered with stomach content.

I was told they were able to push the tube through and it was thought to be inflammation possibly caused by a blood pocket or "something of that nature."

Friday, November 10, 1995

This morning they took me for a CAT scan and asked me to drink some stuff. Again, I explained that I could take very little. The test confirmed where the blockage was, but not what caused it.

By now Ken and I were at the point of "giving up." This couldn't be happening after we had been so positive that the surgery would help. "God," I pray, "why is this happening?"

A senior resident explains to us that because the vomit contains bile, the pyloroplasty operation was most likely "okay," although still healing. I was then told I would have to have a tube put through the nose to the stomach again, and a central nutrition line inserted into one of my arteries, as my nutritional levels were dangerously low.

Dr. Benoski then came in and told me if it didn't unblock by itself, he would have to perform surgery again. He explained that he would have to take out the part of the stomach with the problem and connect the small intestine directly to the stomach. At least that was our understanding of the conversation.

After he left, Ken and I were basket cases. We asked to see a counselor. We were told we would not get help, as it was the weekend and our situation was not considered an emergency. We cried and held each other. What could we do? Ken had to leave and I lay there numb and bewildered.

A nurse came in with a student nurse and asked if the student nurse could put down the tube. It would be her first time and she would be supervised. "Remember," she said, "they have to learn somehow." I answered, "At this point it couldn't get much worse," so she should go ahead. She was nervous and just couldn't do anything. After at number of tries, I grabbed her hand and said, "Let me do this!" I took the tube and pushed it down to my stomach myself. With all that I'd been through, tubes that have to be put through the nose are, by far, one of the worst medical procedures; at least I think so!

Saturday, November 11, 1995

I have to admit the tube has stopped me from vomiting and I'm amazed as to how much it pumps out of my stomach. Today I'm to get the central line put in and I'm so scared! It was explained to me that there were risks, such as punctures, infection, etc. You can well imagine, knowing this did not make me feel better.

The procedure was done in my bed. I was frozen near my shoulder but still felt them working. A resident, who was being guided by the Senior Resident, was doing the procedure. I seemed to be lucky that way. I can assure you no one was laughing now. The Senior Resident was new on this floor and very compassionate and professional. The

200

tube was finally in place and then it had to be stitched. He started to sew but there was no freezing left. I wasn't sure which hurt the most, the sewing or the freezing. So, hidden under my cloth, the tears fell. During the procedure my heart was fluttering, but I was told that was normal.

The nurses then put in all the lines and started feeding me. It seemed that I had tubes everywhere and numerous bottles hanging from a pole. I looked at all of this and wondered how I got here. I prayed that the blockage would open up and I wouldn't need surgery again, something I felt that I wouldn't be able to cope with.

All through this, Ken and Rachelle were so kind and tried to lift my spirits up.

Sunday, November 12, 1995

The last 5 days have all been the same. The nutrition line is feeding me and my stomach is being pumped. After a few days I stopped losing weight and was able to walk a bit while pushing my pole with its bottles and bags. The doctor told us he hoped the blockage would open on it's own, eliminating the need for another operation. My throat was so sore from the tube; I couldn't wait to get rid of it.

I dream of food, food, food! I'm looking at a plate of pasta. As I go to take a bite, a hand takes the plate away. Then a sandwich and pie go by. I'm floating and trying to grab at the food but can never quite reach it.

At mealtime I smell the food go by and think I'm really losing it if I'm craving hospital food. This is making me appreciate what we take for granted and how eating is a major part of our lives.

Father Russ, a very nice priest, comes to visit and pray. He places his hands on my head and prays that soon my stomach will heal and I will once again be with my family. The tears fall as I hear the words that I have said so many times. Who knows, he may have a closer rapport with God than me. He asked if he could share something with me. He felt strongly that someone might be wishing me ill. If I knew who it might be, he said that I should pray for this person because this person was in turmoil and needed help. I thanked him and told him that I couldn't think of anyone who might wish me harm. If that were the case, I would pray and hope the "curse" would be lifted. After he left, I was stunned for a long time, I had never thought of anything like this. I had been ill for so long, was it possible that someone indeed wished me harm? I would not dwell on this because I couldn't see it as a possibility.

Ken started reflexology (massage) on my feet, especially in the area that stimulated the digestive system. He did this for 2 days and I started to bring up dried blood through the stomach tube. On Thursday night Ken and Rachelle put their hands on my stomach and we prayed. We believe in the power of prayer. Maybe we simply were not praying hard enough.

Friday, November 17, 1995

The doctor felt it might be a good idea to try a barium swallow and another x-ray to see if anything was opening up. If the barium didn't go through, it would be pumped out. That morning I felt some movement in my tummy and had a little gas. Now you might think that passing gas isn't exciting, but to me it was great! I knew that our prayers were being answered.

I was taken down for the barium swallow and stomach x-ray. Before starting, they took a regular x-ray of my abdomen and discovered that I still had barium from the 8th or 9th. I thought that might be the case as I had a sore right side. Again the barium was caught at the entrance of the large bowel and looked solidified. They decided not to do the test and sent me back to my room. When I got back, I asked the nurse if I should have an enema. I was told that the resident doctor said he'd rather wait and see if it would work its way down. Well, I guess if things started working again, it might.

Saturday, November 18, 1995

The doctor decided I should try clamping the stomach tube for 3-4 hours at a time. The nurse used her stethoscope and could hear faint tummy noises. I had bowel sounds and increased sounds meant things were starting to go through. I was so excited. Every time the nurse heard any sounds, the news went around the ward. I could only keep the tube clamped 3 hours, but it was a start.

My sister Michelle and her husband Ron came for a visit. My sister Terry, from Montreal, called everyday. Ken and Rachelle were here again and must be tired of having to come every day.

Through all of this, Dr. Heart encouraged me and kept a close eye on me. Because he was so caring, he was a good example to any resident doctor. I was fortunate to have him here and looked forward to his visits. His kind smile pulled me out of many slumps.

Sunday, November 19, 1995

Today was about the same, except I kept the tube clamped for 4 hours. The last few days I had been doing visualization. In my mind I would see little workmen shoveling to open my blockage and see the opening getting bigger and bigger. By the end of the day, I could feel some gurgling in the area of the blockage. It was slight, but it was happening. That day I could strongly feel my parents' presence and kept looking towards the chair where I felt they were. When I closed my eyes and dozed, I could feel Mom sitting in the big chair and Dad standing beside her. They were younger, probably in their 50's, and were smiling at me. As always, Rachelle and Ken were here to be with me. I kept telling them that they shouldn't bother coming every day, but my heart would sing when they walked in.

Monday, November 20, 1995

The doctor decides against the barium test and wants to wait now for the reason that bowel sounds have started. That suited me just fine!

That day I kept the tube clamped most of the day. By this afternoon I had increased bowel sounds and was told the tube might come out Tuesday or Wednesday. I was so excited because by now my nose and throat were very sore and when I swallowed my ear hurt. Instead of swallowing I would spit into a Kleenex. At night I would swallow and the pain would wake me.

I felt sorry for myself since I wanted to be Christmas baking and shopping. Like other Christmases, we would all pitch in and it would be wonderful just to be together.

Tuesday, November 21, 1995

Today my son Robert and his dad Ernie, my former husband, drove down from Edmonton to see me. I was surprised and touched that they would take time to come to visit. We had a nice visit and Robert gave me a huge 4-foot high card that my grandsons Daniel and Marc had made. Rachelle stayed with me most of the afternoon.

Last night I kept the tube clamped most of the night and today it has been clamped most of the day. I can hardly swallow it hurts so much.

Tonight I'm exhausted, probably because I stayed up most of the time today. I have to walk to try getting some strength back. I'm worried because the nurse that changed my feed tube last night dropped it on the floor, wiped it, and then reconnected it. Because everything has to be sterile, I'm concerned.

Wednesday, November 22, 1995

This morning the stomach tube was removed. It feels so good not to have it! Shortly after I started feeling warm and was nauseated. As the day progressed, I felt worse and my temperature started to go up. By evening my temperature was high and I was shivering. "I must have the flu, "I thought. The resident was called in during the night and blood work was taken for bacterial infection.

Thursday, November 23, 1995

Today they decided to take out the central feed line in case I had somehow developed an infection. My fever was still high and I was vomiting. I started diarrhea as well and was convinced I had the flu since it was going around. The doctors agreed that it was probably the flu. Now I was concerned that Ken and Rachelle might get sick.

Friday, November 24, 1995

Last night I perspired heavily all night and the nurse helped me change twice. This morning the fever has started going down. I'm put on I.V. because I'm still weak. By the afternoon the nausea and diarrhea have subsided. I'm trying to drink fluids, but not doing too well yet. Deanne was here and I was scared she would catch this stupid flu.

Saturday, November 25, 1995

Today I'm able to get up, but feel really weak. I want to try walking to build up strength but just about fainted, so I head back to bed.

The doctors decide that I should try full fluids. However, they're having trouble relaying this information to the kitchen staff. I keep getting salty broth that nauseates me.

Ken told me that Joanne and Dennis are driving down tomorrow. I can't wait to see them. I wish that Robert had not seen me with all the tubes when he was here. I'm sure the image was not pretty.

It's hard to believe it's only a month until Christmas. I won't be able to make tourtières with Joanne this year. It's a Christmas tradition and it's so much fun. All the special things I like to do at this time of year are on hold. I have to keep thinking positive. Each day I get stronger and better.

Sunday, November 26, 1995

The morning is long—knowing that Joanne and Dennis will be visiting. Rachelle comes around 1 p.m. and plucks my eyebrows. By now I'm looking pretty scary. I'm thin, my lips are dry and cracked, and my hair is a mess. I guess those things are unimportant when a person is so sick. I've lost about 30 pounds and don't want to lose any more. I have no muscle tone in my arms and legs. I think that it's a good sign to be concerned about my appearance. I even look for lipstick and wish I could do more with my hair.

At 2:30 the kids are here and they take me in a wheelchair to the cafeteria. I look around and feel strange to be among so many people. They came down in Dennis' new truck and parked it where I could see it from my window. After leaving here, they were taking Ken out for his birthday, which is on December 1. I tried not to cry but couldn't help it. I wanted so much to go with them. I watched them drive away feeling sorry for myself.

I'm still on broth and juices. Last night I dreamt that I was in a burger place stuffing a plastic box with burgers. I then put it under my arm and was running up the street. Ken was running after me yelling, "Stop, please stop, you can't eat those, you'll get sick." What a crazy dream.

Dr. Benoski told me he was going to a conference until the 29th and if I were released over the weekend he would see me in his office a week later. I knew I wouldn't be out that weekend. The new resident doctor was a lady with a lot of common sense and said we should wait until I could tolerate pureed foods. Dr. Heart, my surgeon's colleague, agreed with this.

Tuesday, November 28, 1995

The last 3 days were spent about the same. Somehow there is a communication problem with the kitchen staff or is it faith intervening that I shouldn't yet have full fluids. I feel that I have to know if I can tolerate pureed foods before leaving. I couldn't bear the thought of having to come back here again—ever! If I had been monitored properly after surgery, then I probably wouldn't be going through this.

Today I talked to the doctor and asked if I could possibly try a little pureed food, since the kitchen somehow wasn't giving me full fluids. Maybe this message would get through to them. She agreed I could give it a try, but only a few bites the first time.

On Tuesday I was given some pureed carrots and potatoes and even some gravy. I sat there looking at it for the longest time. For the first time I truly knew what a starving person would feel when given food. As I looked at the plate of what seemed to be an enormous amount of food, I cried and asked God to help me digest it. After 6 weeks of not eating, this would be quite an experience. I picked up the fork and didn't know if my first bite would be carrots, no, maybe potato. Yes, I'd go with the potato. I was crying and laughing and wished Ken and the kids were here to share this moment. Food—truly a gift to life, as I now saw it. I took a bite of potato and never has a bite of potato tasted like this. Never again will it taste like that bite. I savored it in my mouth for as long as I could and there I did it, it was swallowed. By this time I was crying so much that I could hardly swallow. I told myself to calm down, relax and pretend this was a banquet. Then came that bite of carrots. Oh, the taste and sweetness! I managed to eat about a half of the carrots and potatoes, about a half-cup in all. I felt like I'd eaten a huge steak. For a time my stomach wondered what was happening. But eventually, I had digested it all and felt like a child at Christmas.

In the evening Father Russ came by and was thrilled to hear I was improving and we said prayers of thanks together. I called Ken and Rachelle and told them that I had eaten!

Wednesday, November 29, 1995

This morning my tray had cream of wheat and pureed peaches. With relish I ate about half, but by mid-morning I wasn't feeling that well and thought it might be the milk or the porridge.

At lunch I ate a little pureed soup and that seemed to go down a bit better. For supper, I had some pureed sweet potato, meat and custard. Oh, the sweet tastes of food! I couldn't take more than one bite of meat and I ate about half of the rest.

The evening brought visitors and after that Ken and I watched TV and played cards. I felt quite well during the evening, but a bit bloated at bedtime. After some Ginger Ale I felt much better.

Dr. Heart came by; he rarely misses a day. He is more like a friend and will be the only one that I'll miss when I leave this place. Dr. Benoski came by later in the evening and was glad that I was on pureed foods. He felt it might be a good idea to have an upper GI barium test to confirm things were functioning okay before I left. I reminded him that the barium drink was liquid and did he think it would confirm how the food was digesting. He told me it would show the opening and give information. I knew I'd have to have this test, but I'm so tired of tests and afraid the barium will get lodged in my bowels again.

By the sounds of it now, I don't know if I'll be home for Ken's birthday. What a bummer that would be! That night I prayed for support and asked God to fill me with the Holy Spirit, his love and healing grace. We had always prayed for the oppressed people in a general sense, and have a World Vision child, but I now had a special prayer added for the sick and hungry people of our world.

Thursday, November 30, 1995

By now I had hoped to be home. Better to stay an extra day or so, than having to come back. The Cream of Wheat didn't sit well with me so I wouldn't eat any more for now. Looking out the window, as I did often, I could see people, cars, houses, and children and felt again detached from this world. I visualized myself in my kitchen baking Ken's birthday cake. I've always enjoyed making birthday cakes for special people. It's a time where I think of the special things that we've shared and how they have enriched my life.

Dr. Benoski and the lady resident felt it would be best to have an upper GI barium test tomorrow to see exactly what was happening. We discussed the possibility of my leaving after, if everything looked okay. I was elated after they left. Tomorrow I might be home and away from this room, doctors and the smell of a hospital.

Rachelle stopped by before doing her student teaching. I try to express how grateful I am for her time with me. She hugs me again and assures me she loves me and is so grateful I'm coming home soon. We hold each other and cry. I watch her leave and I'm so grateful for her love, help and understanding at such a young age.

I'm eating my pureed foods and they seem to be going through my digestive system. At times the pyloroplasty operation site still hurts after I eat. I imagine that all the vomiting has not helped and hope time will heal everything. I'm so grateful that there is improvement and I'm sure the power of prayer has helped. It was a long evening thinking about the test tomorrow and hoping it would be my last night here.

Friday, December 1, 1995

Today is Ken's 47th birthday. These are the times when I find it especially hard to be sick. He told me the best gift he could have, would be to bring me home today.

At 9:00 a.m. I went down for the upper gastro test. It was a follow through to the small bowel, so it took 2 hours in all.

At about 2:00 p.m. the resident came in and said the test showed the barium going through. It had taken a little longer going through the second blockage site, but had gone through. She felt I could go home and would get confirmation from Dr. Benoski. When she told me I could leave, I cried. She said she understood, after all that had happened and the length of time I had been there.

Dr. Heart came to say goodbye. I thanked him for being the person he is, for watching over me and lifting my spirits through this horrible time in my life. I would miss him, but felt too shy to share it with him.

While I waited for Ken to pick me up at 7:00 p.m., I thought of all the people I had met at the hospital and said

211

a prayer that they would be healed. Especially for Mark, who at a young age had a major portion of his bowels removed because of Chrons, and the other man who had most of his tongue removed because of cancer caused by a tobacco habit.

None of my children smoked, but after seeing these things I vowed I would try to stop them if they did.

I put my clothes on to go home and was shaking because I was still so weak. The total inactivity had made my muscles hurt less because chronic fatigue/fibromyalgia always seemed worse for me with activity. The loss of weight and muscle tone was mind-boggling. My pants and sweater hung on me. I told myself to quit bitching about it. I'd always wanted to be thin. I combed my hair, put on lipstick and felt more human than I had for a long time.

Ken picked me up and home we went. It felt so odd being home. I looked around and things seemed so colorful and beautiful. Rachelle hugs me and we laugh and cry.

December 4, 1995

It's so nice to be home! I've been eating pureed foods and very small portions at a time. I'll most likely be on them for a few weeks, but I don't mind as long as things gradually improve.

As I stand at the window watching Ken put up the Christmas lights, I feel so blessed that I've survived. This year there will be some bought baking for Christmas, but together we'll make butter tarts and minced meat tarts, as it's not Christmas without them.

December 25, 1995

Christmas comes and I sit in church for the beautiful service celebrating Christ's birth. My husband and children are with me and it's hard not to cry, as I thank God for geting us through yet another nightmare. I ask for strength and help to cope with this chronic disease and know he will hold my hand when things get rough. My children and husband look at me, smile and my heart sings because I love them so much and I am alive.

STORMS END

It now seems endless, the hurt, pain and despair,
At times, it renders me mindless, impossible to bear.
The world around seems black; I grasp a hand to hold,
To hear, "Don't look back," I need to be told.
I am angry, I want to cry, someone holds me tight,
I feel loved and heave a sigh, hold me into the night.
The rumble in my heart ceases, calming my mind,
A rainbow, the sunshine, the storm is behind.

Annette Stremecki

The following is something a friend sent to me a few years ago. The author is unknown to me and I'm grateful for the use of it. It depicts this disease in a nutshell. Read on...

THE THIEF OF MANY LIVES

I am constantly on the prowl in search of new victims. I do not discriminate when choosing my victims: Health Care workers, teachers, students, airline personnel, moms, dads, anyone is my prey. If you are dynamic and have a lust for life, I will seek you out, and I WILL find you.

Just when you are at the peak of your endeavors, climbing the career ladder or building your family and home, I WILL find you. There is nothing you have in your life that I am not capable of destroying tomorrow: your career, your education, your goals and your dreams, your family and your life. I will have it all. I will strip you of your ability to function at any level above minimal, and from this day on, you will refer to that minimal as a "good day."

I have the ability to create an invalid out of you overnight, and I WILL. It will take a marathon effort for you just to get out of bed. At a cellular level, your immune system will be a constant war battling itself and unnamed viruses, which will painfully be replicating in your brain. I promise you I WILL bring you despair along with pain, isolation and losses far beyond what you can imagine.

Your mind will be in a constant fogged state, your expression will be unable to express, and your eyes will have a noticeable "glazed over" look. You will find it most difficult to pay attention, concentrate or even process the simplest thoughts. Making change from a dollar may even be beyond your ability at times. Your mouth may feel like it's full of marbles when you try to speak, as your tongue twists and nothing you try to say comes out right. Who would believe your level of education when you can't even string enough words together to make a complete sentence... or, one that makes any sense at all?

I promise, I WILL bring you, at an unsuspecting time, severe abdominal pain, nausea, vomiting and diarrhea along with a host of gastro-intestinal disorders. I will make you weak, lifeless, as one could be without being confirmed dead. You will be housebound or in bed for several years if not for the rest of your life. As part of incapacitating you, your heart will race and your head pound: your throat will be sore and you lymph glands swollen. That will all be trivial after I inflame and spasm muscles throughout your body. Crushing a grape between your fingers may take too much energy or be too painful now. Pouring tea from a teapot will be a thing of the past.

On those nights that I allow you to sleep, you will awaken drenched with sweat or throbbing pain. Perhaps, I might even throw in a little seizure activity. On those nights that I do not allow sleep to occur, I WILL torture you with thoughts of death. Not suicide, but death. Simply because you have intermittent numbness and tingling, which resembles an electric current zapping you from time to time. This is called neuropathy. Nope, it doesn't seem curable either.

Now I have you. I have taken over your body and your mind. I have stolen your life but left you alive, not very functional, but by clinical definition, you are still alive!

Your family will not be able to give you the constant care that you need on a daily basis. As for your friends, well, they're still on that ladder climbing up. I am looking for them also. By now, chances are that most of your family and friends have abandoned you, so you must have learned the definition of ISOLATION. This newfound isolation will save you from having to explain how sick you are to others because they won't understand anyway. Isolation will save you all that energy.

Your health insurance has already been or shortly will be discontinued (if you were lucky enough to get some in the first place), as you have most likely lost your job from not being able to "keep up." Perhaps you have called in sick once too often. Now that you are no longer employable or insurable, when you seek medical care, any professional that figures me out, will diagnose you and say that they do not know what you have or, you really aren't sick or, what you have is not curable.

Now you may even try to seek medical care worldwide. However, most medical professionals will not have the ability to recognize me when they see me, as they have not learned about me in medical school. So, chances are that you will be misdiagnosed. You will give more blood samples and have more examinations that you ever imagined possible. Then you can take the results to a dozen doctors in search of help and a diagnosis. One that is valid and medically acceptable. One that does not label you as depressed or say that you are a hypochondriac! Most doctors will suggest a vacation, weight loss, psychological assessment, help with the children, etc. as the cure, mainly because, you may at times look like the picture of health. This is my mask of deception!

You will pray for a positive word from current research. Research, which you will soon learn, is quite limited due to lack of funding and government support. You will learn new vocabulary which contains words like t-cells, cytokines, nuclear antigens, natural killer cells, immunoglobulins, cytomegalovirus, seratonins, cerebral lesions, immune dysfunctions will be amongst a few. However, the most important words that you will need to know and fight for are: Disability Assistance Plans.

At one point I may give you a false sense of recovery or remission. Let me assure you, I WILL be back. I have changed the lives of millions of people worldwide. I now consider myself an epidemic, don't you?

Eventually, I will bring the government, Health Care workers, and society to its knees in search of unraveling my complexities, which are crippling humanity. I leave it up to you, my victims and caregivers to educate the public and let them know I am very real and you are very sick when you succumb to me. There is more and more talk of natural ways of making you function better and even maybe curing you! That is a little unnerving for me. One day I might be a thing of the past, but until then, or until my names are changed, I am...

Chronic Fatigue, and Immune Dysfunction Syndrome, Fibromyalgia.

EPILOGUE

In 1999 Joanne and Dennis had a beautiful son, who they named Nicolas. We again were blessed when their second son Luc was born in 2002.

Also, in 1999 we reapplied for disability benefits under Canada Pension. I had previously applied in 1992, but was rejected. At that time, we were too physically, emotionally and financially drained to continue pursuing the matter. In 2004, with the assistance of a lawyer, my case was brought before an Appeal Panel. After several years of frustration and tiresome exchange, the ruling was in our favor. After all was said and done, the amount we received was rather insignificant, but nevertheless it was a victory worth celebrating. Not only was chronic fatigue/fibromyalgia accepted as a disability in my case, but there was also an acknowledgement that I was disabled in 1992.

In 2004 we celebrated Rachelle and Jed's wedding. I was thrilled to have been given the ability to cope during this special time. In the fall of 2004 I had another relapse but again climbed back up the ladder. In 2005 we rejoiced over the birth of our sixth beautiful grandchild; our first granddaughter, named Tahlia. On May 12, 2008 we were given the gift of another grandson, named Cayden.

It is the summer of 2008 and I am pleased to share that my disease is under control, giving us our life back again. The really bad nightmares are in the background where I hope they will stay. At the age of 66, I have come to the realization that indeed life has its continued challenges. I know I will have relapses and I will cope with them. I continue all the good things I have learned. Through my challenges, I have been taught that age and experience brings strength, skills and wisdom that helped me to cope and heal.

Each day brings with it both the light and the dark. When dark shadows overpower, I tell myself that I'm now better equipped to deal with it. I still find it simply amazing that with help, love and faith we humans have the capability to heal from severe physical and psychological trauma. The opportunity to walk in someone else's shoes has made my spirit fuller, richer and deeper. I am so grateful for the good things and for still being alive!

Chronic Fatigue/Fibromyalgia is finally recognized, but not always accepted within the medical community. Public knowledge of this disease was minimal until 1990. However, there are many more questions to be answered.

I call this disease a modern day disease because more and more people are afflicted. It is also a closet disease because, at times, there are no physical signs. This disease is complex; the symptoms flare up and can mimic other diseases. The pain and fatigue rarely, if ever, totally disappear. What caused me to become so ill? Was it post-viral, toxins? No one can point a finger as to exactly what causes this debilitating disease, but it does exist.

Unfortunately, we live in a world of toxins and pollutants! We are bombarded by emissions from technology. Toxins are in our atmosphere, in our food and drink, etc. Pesticides and herbicides are deadly. We have to fight to stop the use of these toxins for the sake of ourselves, and our future generations. Our bodies are not made to handle

219

such amounts of toxins, thus resulting in numerous diseases.

PREVENTION is the big word to remember. Please be aware, read your labels, quit smoking, reduce your stress level, and help yourself by going organic, if possible. Now, I never purchase anything without reading the label first. Aspartame is a big no in our home, as is anything with preservatives, coloring, etc. We try hard to exclude these from our diet. I can't believe that color is added to so many things. Popcorn??? Give me a break! No need for it! Take your supplements. In the world we live in, they are necessary to survive and keep away disease. Our food doesn't have the nutrition that it had in our grandparents' day. Drink good clean water... lots of it. Your many cups of coffee don't count as they only dehydrate you even more. So savor that one cup of morning coffee. Most people are unaware that they are dehydrated. Have a headache? Drink a tall glass of water; it will most likely cure it within a few minutes.

When you can walk, walk. It is so beneficial and a change of scenery helps. I can't share with you enough how I now appreciate even a short walk! Self-help doesn't have to be expensive. Take some quiet time for yourself; meditate, pray, do yoga or whatever relaxes you. Take time for a long soak and listen to relaxing music. Practice smiling and you'll be surprised at the results.

Chronic fatigue/fibromyalgia will change the level of your performance; your self-esteem will suffer. It's so important to find self-worth in other ways. Everyone is special and we must dwell on our given gifts. It is often hard for your family and friends to understand why you are not the same person or that chronic fatigue/fibromyalgia can be so disabling.

If you have this disorder or think you might, I strongly recommend that you become informed through literature available at your library, health stores, and appropriate support organizations. Seek good doctors who are sympathetic and informed about this disease. Include a naturopathic medical doctor, if possible. They have double the knowledge.

Family, friends, good books and/or counselors are essential to help you cope. These will see you through the rough times. It is especially hard when you're also coping with other medical or emotional situations. So, grab God's hand and accept help when you need it.

Remember, get help and focus on the positive. It might rain on your parade, but life is still a parade. It is your choice to improve the quality of your life. It is your spirit and body to love!

God bless.

Annette Stremecki

ISBN 142517021-8